How to Be a
Bad Bitch

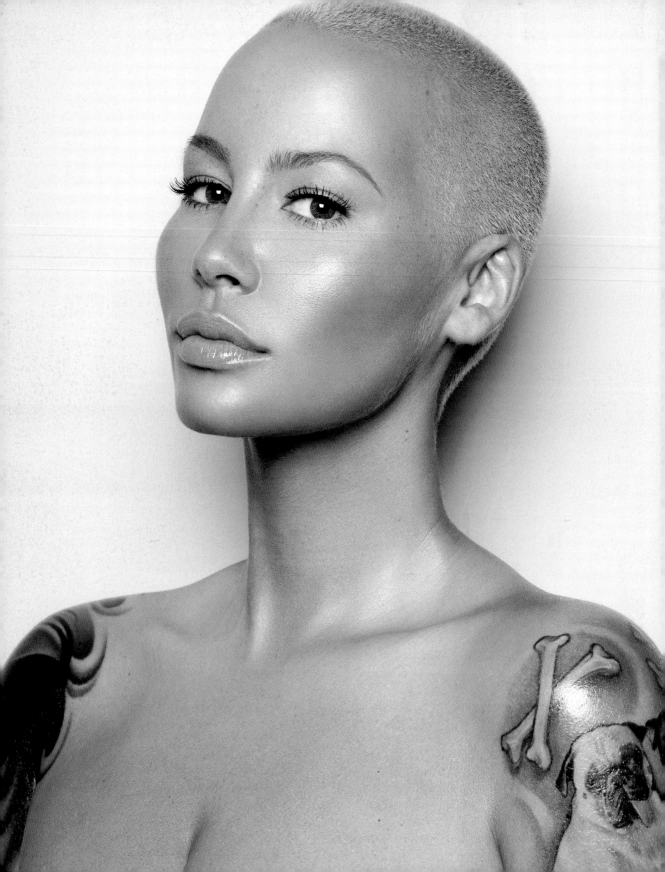

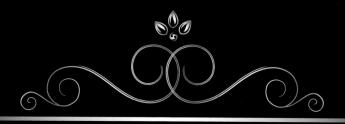

How to Be a
Bad Bitch

Amber Rose

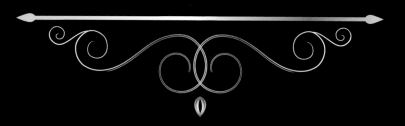

GALLERY BOOKS

NEW YORK LONDON TORONTO SYDNEY NEW DELHI

Gallery Books
An Imprint of Simon & Schuster, Inc.
1230 Avenue of the Americas
New York, NY 10020

First Gallery Books hardcover edition October 2015

GALLERY BOOKS and colophon are registered trademarks of Simon & Schuster, Inc.

For information about special discounts for bulk purchases, please contact Simon & Schuster Special Sales at 1-866-506-1949 or business@simonandschuster.com.

The Simon & Schuster Speakers Bureau can bring authors to your live event. For more information or to book an event, contact the Simon & Schuster Speakers Bureau at 1-866-248-3049 or visit our website at www.simonspeakers.com.

Interior design by Jaime Putorti
Jacket photographs and design by David LaChapelle

Manufactured in the United States of America

10 9 8 7 6 5 4 3 2 1

Library of Congress Cataloging-in-Publication Data is available.

ISBN 978-1-5011-1011-5
ISBN 978-1-5011-1014-6 (ebook)

This book is dedicated to my mom, *Dottie*,

for giving me my confidence, not judging me for my mistakes

in life, and always having my back.

Love you, Mommy.

CONTENTS

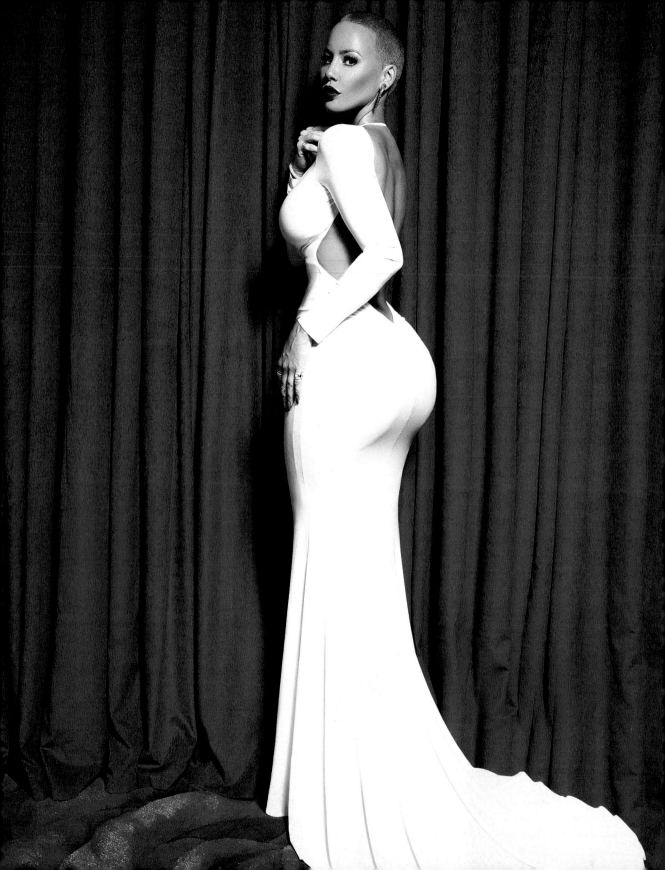

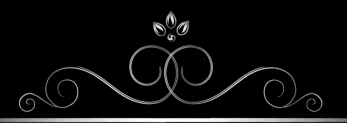

INTRODUCTION

Definition of a Bad Bitch

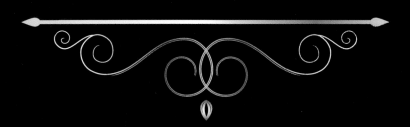

I'm writing this book because I decided to do something for myself, no fucks given. And so here I am, telling my story, as a way to help all of you become the best you can be. I've got plenty to tell, and plenty of advice to offer, having faced all kinds of trials and tribulations during every stage of my life. I've learned from hard experience: pain eventually turns into strength.

But first things first. You might be surprised to learn that being a bad bitch doesn't mean acting like a bitch at all. Sure, a bad bitch puts herself first—she has the vision to create her own unique look and devotes the time and energy to take care of herself and be well put together—always. But she also takes her obligations seriously—to work, her family, her friends, and, when she chooses to have a man, him, too—and she shows up when she says she will. She has impeccable manners, no matter what. She can afford to be generous, in word and deed, because she knows she's got plenty of everything she needs. She's together and strong in body, mind, attitude, and finances. She gets what she wants by any means necessary. When things don't go the way she wants them to, she takes the time to grieve her loss, learn the lessons to be learned, and come back a badder bitch than ever.

I was born a bad bitch. Even when my mom was raising me on a waitress's salary in South Philly and kids were calling me Four Eyes. Even when I became an exotic dancer. Even when I got myself to New York at twenty-one and lived on nothing, I knew I had it, and I've never lost sight of that. Along the way, I kept my eyes open and gained experience wherever I could, and that's also how I came to be the Muva of all my fans, my Rosebuds. Not to say I haven't made my fair share of mistakes over the years. In many ways, this book is a collection of all my errors in judgment and all the lessons I've had to learn the hard way, so that maybe you can sidestep the setbacks I've faced. But even when I was down and out, I knew I'd be on my way back up soon, and I always knew I was a bad bitch. Which is the gift I want to give you. Because you've got it, too. You do. So here it is, the handbook to teach you how to be a bad bitch in all aspects of your life.

Being a bad bitch doesn't mean acting like a bitch at all.

Let's get it done.

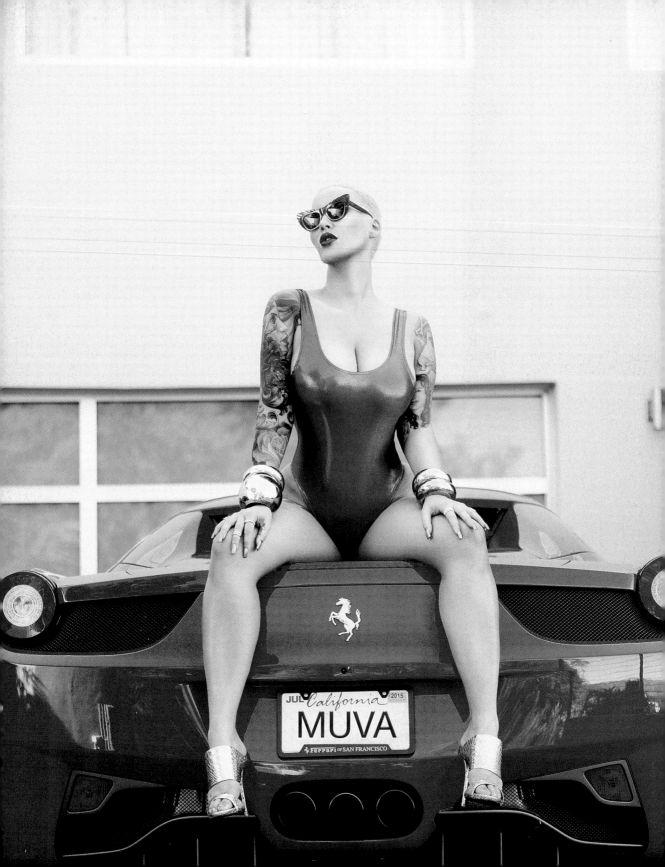

1
VISION

A bad bitch is the mistress of her reality. This means formulating a vision of who you are and what you want, and then taking the necessary steps until you have it all. No matter how crazy your dream may seem to everyone else. Who cares what they think? A bad bitch is not in the business of pleasing other people, thank you very much.

Take South Philly, for example. I'm proud as hell to be from there, and so much of my strength comes from my experiences growing up. But I always had this feeling of not quite being at home there. As much as I loved my friends, we had very different visions of our futures. I swear to God, on my life, that I always used to say to my friends: "I don't belong here. This city is too small for me. I'm going to live in Hollywood."

My friends didn't get it. Not even my childhood friend Monique. Our moms knew each other, too, and both were raising us alone on their waitress salaries, but her mom was a functioning crack addict, and my mom's biggest vice was her cigarettes.

Once when we were twelve, we were having a snack after school at the diner where my mom worked because we could eat there for free.

"I want to have a baby," Monique said.

Now, I knew what sex was, but I certainly hadn't had any. I was a late bloomer, especially by my neighborhood's standards, and I still played with dolls.

"Why would you want to have a baby?" I said. "That's crazy."

"I met this guy, and I want to have a baby with him," she said.

"Girl, you have your whole life in front of you," I said. "If you do that, you'll be stuck in Philly for the rest of your life. Don't you want to get out of here?"

"Amber, my mom's on crack, and my dad's an alcoholic," she said. "At least if I have a baby, it'll show me love, and I'll be happy."

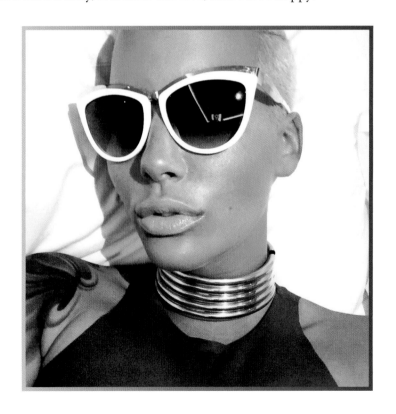

"Well, look, I'm not going to be here for the rest of my life," I said. "I'm going to move to Hollywood, and I'm going to get my mom out of Philly."

"You live in a one-bedroom apartment with your mom. You're never going to live in Hollywood," she said.

It wasn't just Monique who said this stuff to me, and I heard them. I knew they were right, from their perspective. There was absolutely nothing in my day-to-day life to indicate I'd ever find a way out or end up anywhere better. And yet I really, truly believed in my heart that there was no way I was going to be stuck in Philly forever—even when Monique did get pregnant in middle school, just like she'd said she would.

See, I grew up a regular girl, with no status or connections or anything else to get me started. And still, I knew I was going to be a model, and I was going to live in Hollywood. And that's exactly what happened.

But how did I do it? The same way a bad bitch does everything else: with vision.

BEING A BAD BITCH IS A STATE OF MIND

I created an ideal vision of myself, for myself. I put it together, and I pursued it relentlessly. Of course, this was long before *The Secret,* that book that says if you really believe in something, it can happen. But it was just like that. I really believed I was going to end up in Hollywood. And even though there were almost no show business opportunities in Philadelphia, I made the most of every one that came my way. I learned that it pays to be professional and sweet at the same time. You don't have to be so professional that you're a bitch. You have to work your charm.

Take how I got my first modeling gig in Philadelphia. My mom had raised me to have good manners, and on top of that, I was always kind of upbeat and nice to basically everybody I met. Between that and my unique style, which we'll get to in the next chapter, everyone in our neighborhood knew who I was. That's why, when I was still in high school, I got asked by a friend of a friend to do a spring fashion segment for the local television news. It wasn't like I had any modeling experience or media training, but they thought of me as a cool girl who'd be good at that type of lifestyle reporting. So just like that, I got to be on TV, which was amazing, because everyone in Philly watched the news back then, so it was a big deal. And because I believed in myself and had the vision to see my future success, I did well on the show. Sure, it was only a one-off thing, but it gave me confidence. And after that, I could always say I had modeling and TV experience, because I did.

I created an ideal vision of myself, for myself. I put it together, and I pursued it relentlessly.

At that time, in Philly and New York, there was a fabulous gay ballroom scene with rival "houses," each named for a fashion designer. When

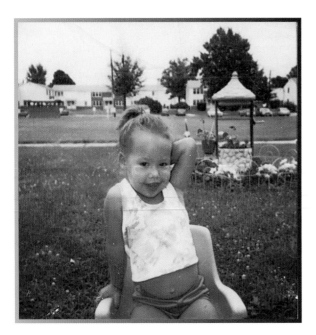

Two years old in Fort Dix. I'd been eating a blue Popsicle when my mom said, "Pose for me, baby." And I gave her that. I still do that pose.

I was in high school, my friend Maurice and I ran into this older gay guy, John Karan, who was the father of the House of Donna Karan in Philadelphia. "I love your face," he said to me in his thick East Coast accent. "You're my dawta, and I'm your fava, and we're going to have you walking face in the balls." I knew that balls were underground competitions where women went up against each other in categories like skin, teeth, and face structure, or "face." Now, I'm against the idea of women being judged against each other, or even compared to each other, but at the time I was still growing into my understanding of what a bad bitch was, and besides, I knew the competition wasn't mean-spirited. It was meant to be flamboyant and fabulous. And I was always into trying something new.

"All right, I guess," I said.

It was *so much fun*. I loved it. I learned so much about style from that whole world, which was really all about being a bad bitch in your own show-stopping way. Well, every house in the ballroom scene had a Fava, Muva, Sista, and Brotha (or that's what it sounded like because of everyone's thick Philly accent). At the time, I was a baby compared with everyone else, so I was Dawta. But when I grew up into a bad bitch with so many incredible fans, all my Rosebuds, I decided to be your Muva. I really feel that way about all of you. You're all my babies, and I want to help you be happy, successful, and fulfilled. I want to help you be the baddest bitches ever.

A True Vision Isn't Fleeting

I always kept my vision crystal-clear in my head, no matter how far it seemed from my reality. And so, when I became an exotic dancer, I didn't worry that it was going to be my life forever. I don't have any sob stories about bad things that happened to me then. It was an honest, fun job, and I loved it. I danced onstage, made my money, and went home to pay my bills. And along the way, I learned so many lessons that I still draw on today.

And even though when I first left Philly at age twenty-one I wasn't quite ready to move to Hollywood, I didn't let the delay worry me. I only had the money to move to New York City, but I knew my next destination would be Hollywood. And three years later, it was.

When I got ready to leave for New York, I had no plan. I just knew that God didn't want me in Philly, for sure. I knew I didn't belong. I envisioned myself being somewhere else, and I always really believed it. I wasn't scared to get the hell out of my hometown, like a lot of people are. I knew that I didn't want to be getting pregnant in high school, getting married to the neighborhood guy, wasting my life away, and not traveling the world and doing everything I wanted to do. Not that there's anything wrong with that, of course. If that's ultimately what you want in life, then that's what you should do. But for me, that was not what I wanted at all.

Let me tell you, this was a moment when there were more people than ever telling me how wrong I was to dream as big as I was dreaming. Especially the guys I was dating, who knew deep down inside they were never getting out of Philly. They certainly didn't want some bitch rubbing it in by leaving them behind. I really cared about one guy, but he already had two kids, and he wasn't going anywhere soon. I was always clear on the fact that I knew who I was, and they didn't. Never let a man's insecurity—or anyone's insecurity—rob you of the vision you have of yourself.

BELIEVING IS ACHIEVING

There were many times when I was uncertain, and I didn't know how I would make all my dreams come true. But I always absolutely believed that somehow, someday, I would. Again and again, I said to myself, *When the next step in your vision happens, it will just happen, and you'll figure it out as you go.*

That's exactly what I did. Let me tell you, it was not glamorous. When I first moved to New York, I lived in the projects in the Bronx. But I didn't let that worry me. I knew it wasn't going to be the end-all-be-all for me. I just had to take an initial step to get the hell out of where I was, and that was it. There were times when it was really scary. I was in New York, I didn't know many people, and it was kind of lonely.

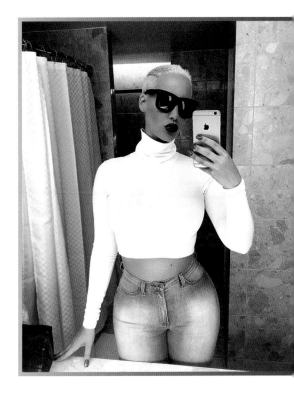

I got a job as an exotic dancer in Mount Vernon, and I stayed to myself. Not only was dancing how I made my money, but it was a good workout, too. I exercised every day, because I had this vision of myself as a model, and I knew I had to be fit to achieve it. I worked as much as I could, trying to stack up my money. It actually helped not to have many friends, because I wasn't going out much, so I didn't have to spend a lot of money. I was essentially saving everything I earned.

I was determined to make it as a model, but I didn't have any connections in New York, so I offered to model for clothing stores in my neighborhood. They didn't really pay me, and the exposure wasn't honestly that great. But it was more experience, and I knew it'd only be a matter of time before my big break. And soon enough I was discovered, which we'll get to in a bit. So that's what it really comes down to: believing is achieving.

FIGURE OUT WHO THIS BITCH IS

First things first: to have a vision of yourself, you've gotta figure out who you are. Maybe you know. Maybe you've always known. If so, more power to you. If not, dare to experiment with different visions before finding your authentic self and path. Be really honest with yourself. If you love to read and write, even if no one else in your family or community does,

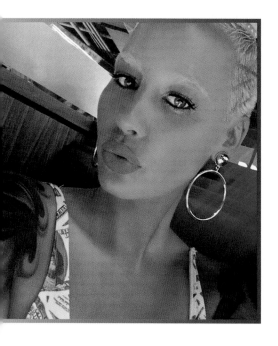

embrace your truth and move toward what feels rewarding for you. The same goes with astrophysics, or interior design, or being a mom. No one but you knows the role you were meant to play in this lifetime. And don't be afraid to make mistakes while you're finding yourself, either. Experimentation is the spice of life, but there's no way every attempt will turn out perfect. Far from it. That's OK. It's how we learn what works for us, and what doesn't, and what's important to us, and what's not.

Don't Worry about Being Normal

Your true vision for creating your ideal self is some version of how I created my life for myself. It's not something that requires money or a diet or a bunch of fashion magazines. It's something you find by looking inside and by taking a risk. I'm telling you now, don't worry about being normal, because you'll just blend. At the core, everyone is perfectly unique and beautiful in her own completely original way. But women are so bombarded with what's "in," or what they "should" do, it can be hard to break free from that mold.

You've gotta give yourself permission to be free, permission to be you. To figure out who you are, dig deep and dare to picture your dream life: where you live, what you do for work, who you love, and who loves you. Lay out the steps required to get there, and then go for it—with everything you've got—until you make it happen.

Who Are You Going to Listen to, Them or You?

It starts with a vision, and that part doesn't have to be hard if you have faith. I think every woman has a vision of her true self and who she wants to be, right? That's why we read the self-help books, and go to the gym, and take

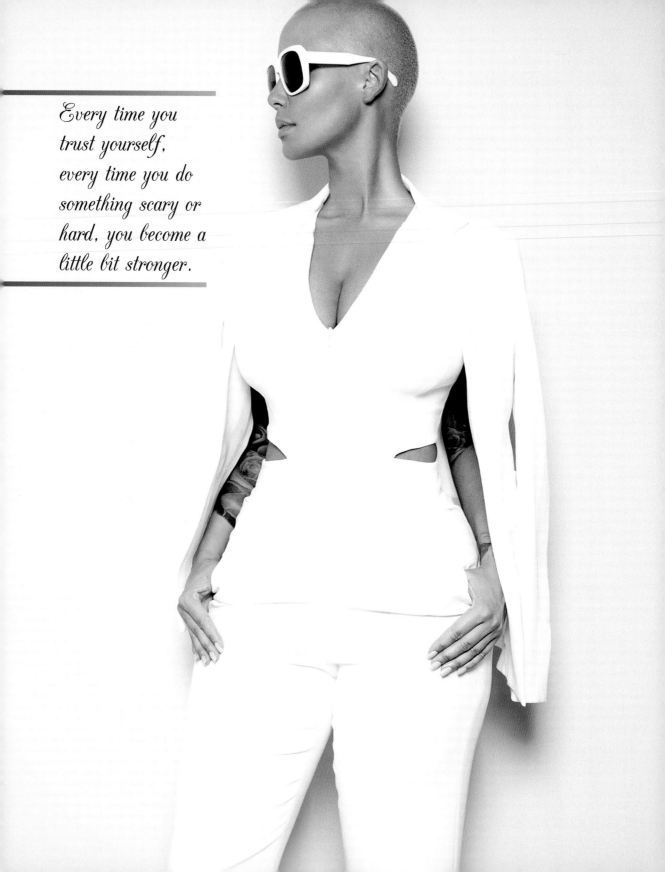

Every time you trust yourself, every time you do something scary or hard, you become a little bit stronger.

the night classes, and talk for hours with our girlfriends about how we're really going to follow our dream this time, because we all want to be a certain way, like we see ourselves in our heads.

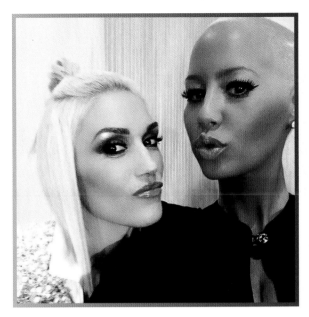

With one of my bad bitch inspirations, Gwen Stefani

In order to execute this vision of yourself, you have to believe, and that's what will give you the confidence you need to go through with your plan and not care what anyone says. Hence my look, my life as a model, my move to Hollywood. Even though no one thought any of it made sense, I knew it was right for me.

Who are you going to listen to, them or you? You only live once. You have to take chances. You have to make your own decisions. You can ask your friends and family for their opinions, but at the end of the day, if you feel very strongly about what you want to do, you should do it.

Others can only tell you what they think, and they're not always right. They're not you. They don't know how it feels to be you. You are the only one who knows who you are and where you're going. Think about it this way: If I'd listened to the people in my life, I'd still be in Philadelphia, and that's not where I'm meant to be at all.

That said, sometimes it's helpful to get advice from somebody you trust. Like me with my manager, Nick. Sometimes he gives me input that guides me. It's important to be clear on your vision and your plan for achieving it, but you also want to have good people around you. And if something's really not working out, you have to be willing to know when to let go and move on to something else.

DON'T WORRY ABOUT HURDLES; THEY WERE MADE TO JUMP OVER

The good news is that every time you take a chance, every time you trust yourself, every time you do something scary or hard, you become a little bit stronger. You become a little bit more of a bad bitch. All you have to do is stay focused. Don't worry about hurdles; they were made to jump over—and offer lessons along the way.

Everything in life is a stepping-stone. You've got to see it that way, no matter how hard it is. My marriage didn't last, but I know it's not the end for me, even though it feels like it sometimes. I know I'm a catch. Sometimes things don't work out, and that doesn't mean it's all your fault. It means you trusted your vision, and that bit of it didn't work out—and that's OK. Something else will. This is just what God wanted.

BUILD YOUR BEST SELF — FROM THE INSIDE OUT

Now that I've helped you to find a vision for creating your best, truest self, I'll show you how you can build on this initial fantasy image of yourself, starting with your appearance (beauty, fashion) and then your manners, your approach to life, and what you care about—from money and friends to sex and a relationship (when the time is right). I'll cover how to come back after you get pushed around and how to evolve, even when life hasn't given you motivation. I'm still doing it today, checking in with myself to make sure I live in the best way I possibly can—even when life doesn't cooperate—and getting myself back on track when I need to. There's something to be said for always staying one step ahead of everyone else. For sure.

And that's how a bad bitch uses her vision to build herself from the inside out. She definitely knows exactly what she wants out of life. She knows what she's not going to deal with. She knows what she's striving for. She's willing to do what it takes to get exactly what she wants, always.

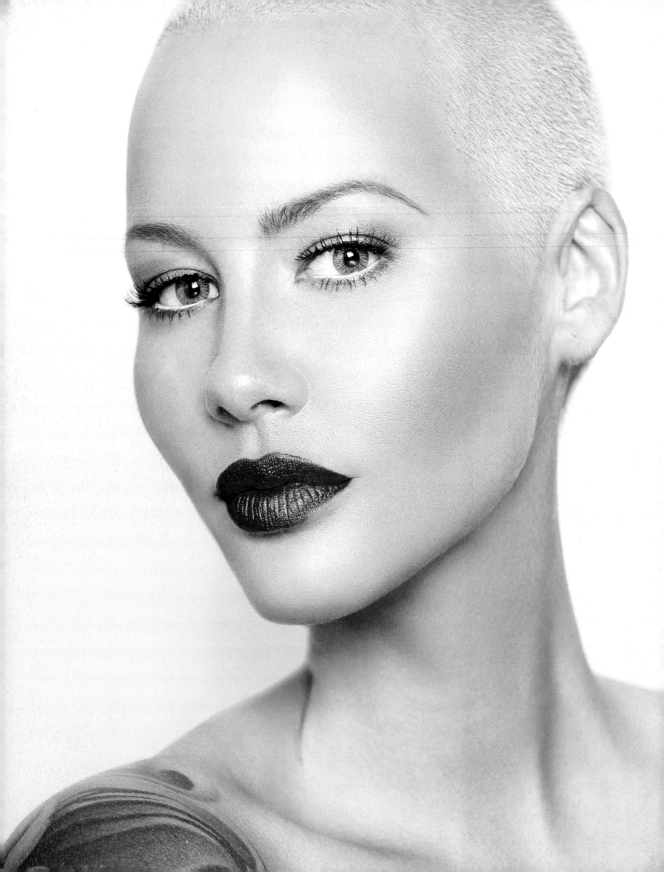

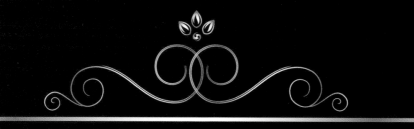

2

BEAUTY

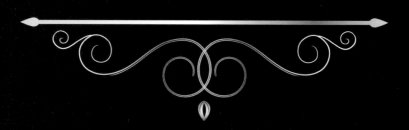

Every woman is born a bad bitch, but I definitely didn't start out looking like one. Although I've always been clear on my vision for my life, there was a time when I didn't really know what I was doing with my appearance. If you don't believe me, because you've seen me in magazines and on the red carpet, you're about to—because I'm gonna spill plenty of embarrassing stories, plus the beauty and fashion truths I came to know the hard way.

TAKE REALLY BIG RISKS

Naturally, my hair grows upward. And then outward. I'm part Cape Verdean and part Italian and Irish, and let me tell you, that equals some curly hair, and not small curls, either, but big curls, like a big, big wave. I guess that could be a pretty intense look if I let it be, but that's never been enough for me. I've always had this drive to really express myself with my hair. Even when I didn't have any money for the salon, I was always experimenting at home.

There was the time I braided my hair. And the time I did the half-braid, hair half out. And the time I added little strands of weave color. And the time I did the Shirley Temple curls with the curling iron, and I mean *really* tight curls. Or the time I put my brown hair up in a ponytail and made two big curls in the front, which I dyed green with Kool-Aid. I know, it may be hard to believe, but this is a real thing. Because I had virgin hair that had never been dyed before, when I coated it in Kool-Aid and wrapped it in tinfoil, my hair soaked up the color and turned bright green.

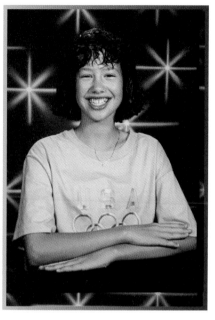

My sixth grade class picture, taken when I was twelve years old and staying with my dad and stepmom in Colorado.

I have a lot of pictures where I look wild. But so what? I mean, for me, at that age, green or blue hair was magic. Truthfully, it still is. I just dyed my hair blue for Easter, and it was a fun look to have for a few days.

There were the total disasters, too, which actually taught me more than the looks I thought were cool. Like the time I cut my bangs myself. I was young and inexperienced, and I didn't realize how much I'd been pulling my hair down to trim it or how much it would spring back when I let go. I stared in the mirror with horror. My bangs were *short*. I looked crazy. *Oh, my God, what did I do?* I hurriedly grabbed my curling iron. There wasn't really much I could do, but I made my bangs into one huge curl. I still looked weird when I went to school, but at least it looked like I'd intended to make it that way.

"What the fuck did you do to your hair, Amber? You look crazy."

I sighed, looking forward to the day when I would live in Hollywood and could look "crazy" without anyone saying anything. For now, though, there was nothing to do but wait for my bangs to grow out.

A few weeks later, I walked into school and saw not just one but two girls with single big curls. That didn't mean I was going to stop growing my bangs in; I did not like how that curl looked on me. But such moments definitely gave me even more confidence to be as extreme as I wanted with my appearance.

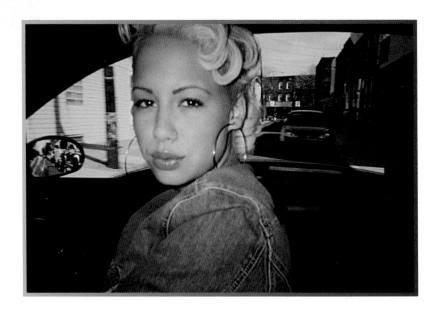

When I was sixteen, I was still experimenting with my hair until I found my look.

When I was sixteen, I had a Mohawk, way before that was cool. Like, I know there was a moment in time when Puff and everyone had a Mohawk, but I did it back when the other kids were looking at me like I was nuts.

And then, when Lil' Kim came out, I wore my hair in all different-colored waves like she did. That was actually cool. But always, I think I was working up to the big one.

When Inspiration Strikes, Go with It

I wanted to shave my head for a long time, but I wasn't sure it was a good idea. So I put my hair in a really tight ponytail, and I looked at my head from the side in the mirror, and I kept thinking, *I don't know if my head shaved will look good enough to really do this.* I asked all of my friends, "Should I shave my head?"

"Amber, you're going to look crazy."

"Don't do it."

"You're going to look stupid as fuck."

I heard them, and of course, they were voicing my worst fears. But I couldn't get the idea out of my mind. I think that's how it is. And since I am rebellious, the fact that everyone thought it was a bad idea just made it more tempting to prove them wrong.

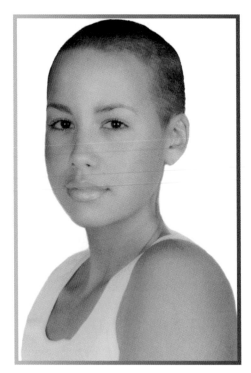

A picture from when I first shaved my head. It's hard to believe that was thirteen years ago! My mom used to carry this picture with her everywhere, even to work.

One morning in 2002, I woke up, and I just knew that was the day.

"You know what . . . I'm going to do it," I said.

I was broke, so I went to the barbershop instead of a salon. I knew what I wanted, but even until the last minute, I was nervous that I wouldn't actually go through with it.

When I sat down in the chair, the barber put the smock over my clothes. I locked eyes with him in the mirror.

"I want you to shave it, and I want you to start straight down the middle so I can't turn back," I said.

As soon as he shaved my head and I saw my reflection, I started to cry. *Oh, my God, I can't believe I just did this to myself,* I thought. It was such a huge difference in my look. And it was such a big deal, especially for a girl, to cut off all her hair, and especially back then. But there was no going back now, and I liked that fact.

My hair is naturally dark, and I left it like that—a brown buzz cut—for maybe a week. I was close to my vision, but I had this nagging sensation that something still wasn't right. And then inspiration struck: *Maybe if I dye my hair blond, it will soften my features a little bit.* I tried it, and I've been buzzed and blond for thirteen years now.

A Bad Bitch Stops Traffic

It was obvious to everyone that I had found my look, no matter how people felt about it. Back in Philly, I stopped traffic. Seriously. I'd be walking down the street, and a car would pull up alongside me, and the window would go down, and out would pop this head, just staring at me. Sometimes it was a man. Sometimes it was a woman. But they always said basically the same thing: "Oh, my God, I've never seen a woman look so beautiful with a shaved head."

I felt that. Here was beauty on my own terms. Here was a look that not only brought out my cheekbones, but also showed off my independence and instantly identified me as a bad bitch. And people got it. They responded to

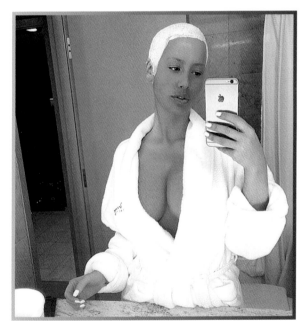

Getting ready for an event in Vegas. Sometimes you gotta bleach on the go.

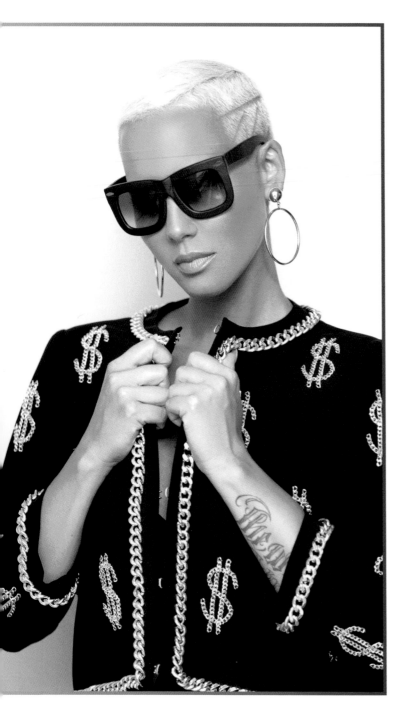

it. Receiving so much positive reinforcement made me feel even stronger and more confident. Rather than making me self-conscious, all of the attention made me blossom. I had so much confidence because I wasn't hiding behind *anything* anymore.

I felt this way even when some people looked at me like I was out of my buzz-cut mind and said things that weren't exactly compliments, like "What made you do that?" Clearly, they weren't into my look, but I never forgot that was just *their* opinion.

It didn't matter to me if no one else knew what they were seeing; I knew who I was. It was like finding my look had helped me find myself, and that set me free. I got all of that from a ten-dollar buzz at the barbershop, the cheapest, easiest haircut there is.

When I think back, this was always my look. And it was exactly what I'd envisioned since I was young. It was exactly what I'd always wanted to look like. I'd finally found the courage to go through with it.

Once I actually acted upon my vision, everything started to fall into place for me. Why? Because I was presenting the most *me* possible. No one could tell me that short hair wasn't happening or curves weren't in, because all they had to do was take one look at me—and how confident and sexy I was—and see it was all working for me. Who was anyone else to argue with results like that?

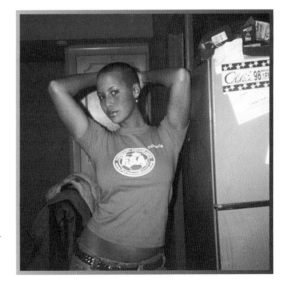

At the little apartment in Philly where my mom and I lived, striking a pose, with my new look. It all started happening for me after that. I dyed my hair blond, and that was that.

IT TAKES COURAGE AND STRENGTH TO BE A BAD BITCH

I always took a cue from the popular girls back in high school, and honestly, they weren't necessarily that cute. Seriously. When I look back, I realize something wild. Dude, I was actually prettier, physically, than most of these girls, but I was a bit introverted, and I wasn't compatible with them. They had so much confidence, and so they got way more attention than I did. That's why everyone loved them and wanted to be around them all the time. It wasn't until I conjured my blond buzz cut that I became self-assured in the same way. And let me tell you what else: they had that clarity of vision to separate out what would work for them and what wouldn't. When those girls looked at a hairstyle in a magazine, they could see it on themselves and think, *No, I can't do that. That's not for me. I will look stupid as hell if I do that.*

I had so much confidence because I wasn't hiding behind <u>anything</u> *anymore.*

Maybe they looked to magazines for ideas and inspiration, but they looked to themselves for what was right, and that positivity just shone out of them. Finally finding my look did that for me, too. The power and confidence it gave me busted all doors open for me and eventually launched my career. Because, finally, I really knew who I was, and I didn't care what anyone else had to say about it, and *that* is hot.

Trust Yourself

Guess what? Remember how all my friends told me I was going to look crazy with my hair buzzed, but I defied the norm and did it anyway? That right there is a bad bitch. You also have that courage and strength inside of you, and you can tap into it, too. You don't need to have money to express yourself. You have *you*, and you know *you* way better than anyone else. You just have to trust yourself and what you know is your true look. You have access to affordable salons. Hell, barbershops are cool, too, and they're *cheap*. If you're too broke even for that, there are people in your neighborhood who know how to do something really great. I guarantee it. Nowadays, with the Internet, you can even look up tutorials for hair and learn how to do it yourself, instead of paying someone. If you see an idea in your head and you know it's you, give it a try. It can't hurt. It could change everything. It did for me.

Let me tell you, I'm all for challenging boring definitions of normality and making a conscious effort to create a unique look for yourself. But that doesn't mean falling prey to the clownish look that can result from not knowing the basics. And you should always make sure you look presentable, even just for going to the corner store. You never know who you're going to run into. Fear not, though. It's really not hard. And I've got your back, girl. I learned by trial and error, so you don't have to.

DON'T FOLLOW TRENDS IF THEY DON'T LOOK GOOD ON YOU

For starters, the first lipstick I wore, when I was twelve or thirteen, was a really dark liner with a light brown lipstick. Now, in my defense, this was back in the day, when that was the cool look everyone was going for. But does that mean it actually looked good on me? Hell, no. It made me look ridiculous. That's why I always say it's better to rock what actually suits you, rather than what everyone else is doing just because it's "in." Don't follow trends if they don't look good on you. Dare to think for yourself and be honest about what you see in the mirror. If it ain't working, it ain't working.

Just as important: learn the basics. Even when I made slightly better choices on the makeup front, it took me a while to have any idea what I was doing. When I really became a bad bitch, I learned to use all the essentials that create a polished look, whether I'm going for more of a natural appearance or full-on glamazon for the red car-

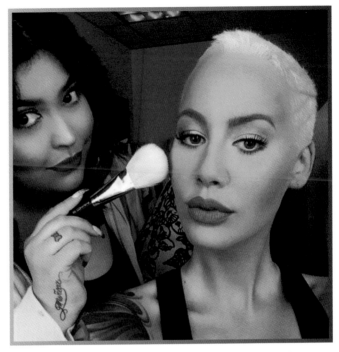

Getting ready with Priscilla, the best makeup artist in the world, and my best friend.

pet. There are many steps involved, and they all happen in a particular order. That's how you put it together. It's like a painting. I also learned some pro shortcuts for days when I don't have time to create my full look. For example, statement sunglasses are an easy fix if you're not able to do your eye makeup. They can also make your outfit pop.

Lucky for me, I have Priscilla Ono in my arsenal. She first did my makeup for a Smirnoff commercial and print ad four years ago. We've been besties ever since. Not only did I love the way she made me look, but I also loved the way she made me feel. Priscilla already ruled on the makeup front, and she taught me her ways.

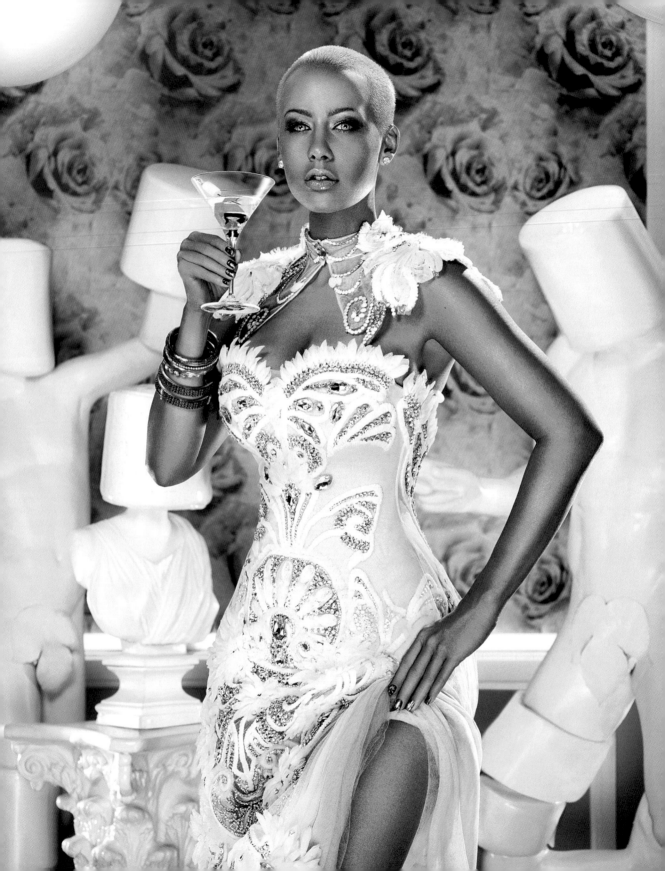

Priscilla is a gold star bad bitch, and she's also one of the sweetest, most genuine people you're likely to run into, especially in Hollywood, where a lot of wack shit can go down. Seriously, meeting her changed everything for me. Not to say I haven't made my share of beauty mistakes since then—but she's kept right on teaching me, which has made all the difference.

Our friends can be our best resources. Maybe your bestie isn't one of the top makeup artists in the biz like mine is. But I'm sure you can think of one or two of your friends who have already put their looks together. You know the ones I mean—whether they're at an afternoon barbecue or the hottest club, they always look perfect. Don't be afraid to hit up your friends for advice, just like I do with Priscilla. You could come right out and ask them what they do to look their best. And if there's a product or technique you're not familiar with, see if they'd be willing to teach you. Maybe even ask them to look you over and give you an honest assessment of how you could improve your hair and makeup game. As you know, though, I'm all for having you define what looks good for yourself, so if their suggestions don't jibe with how you see yourself, don't do anything to compromise your personal vision. On the other hand, good advice is good advice.

> *Don't follow trends if they don't look good on you. Dare to think for yourself and be honest about what you see in the mirror.*

There's affordable makeup out there, even at your local drugstore, and it can be just as good as pro makeup. If you know how to apply it correctly, you can look perfectly made up for almost no money. Most fashion magazines include makeup recommendations featuring less expensive brands, and there's nothing but free information out there on the Internet. All you have to do is take the time to school yourself in the basics. Plenty of department stores and makeup shops will give you a free consultation, helping you to find the best products and shades for you, and then you can use that knowledge to go wild at the drugstore for way less money.

Once you've stocked your makeup bag, it's time to learn how to use your tools and make yourself over, bad-bitch style. There are a million little

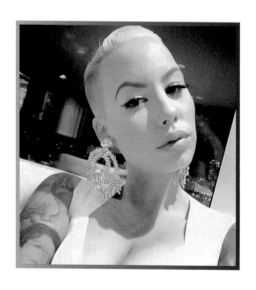

tips. Did you know there are different ways of doing makeup for different face shapes? There are. Once you've looked at a few examples of various women through online tutorials, fashion magazines, and your own group of friends, you'll be able to compare your facial structure with theirs and decide which makeup techniques are right for you.

Then take it step by step. There are magazine articles, books by world-class makeup artists, and online tutorials on how to apply foundation and contour and highlight your face; how to use eye shadow, liquid liner, mascara; the basics for lip liner and lipstick. Plus, there are guides to help you learn how to put it all together. For example, if you're going to do a dramatic eye, always do a lighter lip, and vice versa.

PRACTICE, PRACTICE, PRACTICE

When you're deciding how much makeup you feel comfortable wearing and what look is best for you, remember there's no one right answer. You don't have to put on a ton of makeup—or any makeup at all, for that matter—to be a bad bitch. Attitude and vision are much more important than wearing this season's lipstick trend. But anything and everything you decide to wear should be applied masterfully and with confidence. Even the smallest amount of makeup can make you look like a clown when put on carelessly or without technique.

You've probably heard the saying "practice makes perfect." I mean it: practice, practice, practice. Every single day. Take some time out, park yourself in front of the mirror, and go through the steps provided by your sources—whether they're online instructional videos or your friends— several times. Until you've mastered the essentials: eyebrows, mascara, eye shadow, eyeliner, lashes, foundation, contour, highlights, blush, powder,

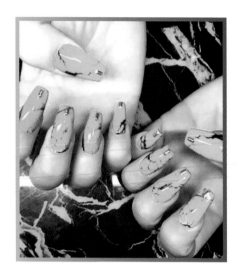

lipstick. I know that may sound like a lot, but the trick is to apply it so it doesn't *look* like a lot. And just because you know how to do all this, that doesn't necessarily mean you're going to wear every component every day. If you do, it's obviously going to look like heavy makeup, and that's a particuar appearance you may or may not be going for. Besides, you probably don't have time to put on false eyelashes before you run to the store or take your kids to school. But the more experienced you are, the more quickly and expertly you'll be able to apply even the slightest accent of mascara and gloss. And when the time comes for you to pull out the big guns—a date, a job interview, a holiday party—you'll be a seasoned pro who can get ready in no time.

If you're prone to breakouts, you need fuller coverage, but even so, there are techniques for making yourself look polished—with just the right colors and contours—not shellacked. You don't want to look like a drag queen, unless you are one, in which case you're already a makeup pro.

Regardless of whether you feel more beautiful in light makeup or looking like you just got a makeup-counter makeover, any techniques you use must be masterful. Remember, the whole point of makeup is to accentuate your natural beauty, to make your eyes look bright and engaged, to make your skin look luminous and fresh, to make your lips look plump and kissable. When used incorrectly, products can actually backfire on you. Lining your entire eye in black can make it appear narrower than it is. While if you use colored eyeliner on your top lash line and apply a white accent at the corners of your eyes, you can easily create the big, beautiful eyes you want. In the same way you wouldn't go into an exam or a big meeting at work unprepared, you don't want to tackle your face without a little knowledge and preparation. That way, you can own every aspect of your look, rather than potentially being a victim of your own beauty limitations. You want to be on point in all areas of your life, right?

DON'T LET YOURSELF LOOK LIKE A CLOWN

As long as you feel your look is representing the true you, go for it. If your technique is masterful, you can rock anything. The truth is, any makeup that's done poorly, no matter how fresh, just looks bad. That's why you practice.

As for lighting, don't do like I did a few years back, before this party I was hosting in Vegas. I was getting ready in a room that was very dim. Even though there wasn't any kind of lighting, I went ahead and did my makeup. I didn't check myself or get a second opinion. I went out to the pool. And I looked like a fucking clown. I mean, my blush was so heavy it was like paint, and my eye makeup was even worse. Every time I come across that picture online, I cringe. Of course, we all make mistakes sometimes, and it's not the end of the world. A bad bitch is all about holding her head high no matter what. But we've all felt how moments like this can really mess with our confidence, and we definitely don't want that. There are enough challenges in life without sabotaging ourselves.

A bad bitch always walks into a room feeling like she owns it, so do everything in your power to make sure you look your best. Taking a little extra time to double-check your look in a mirror, *in proper lighting,* can go a long way. Be your own best friend, and give yourself a long, hard look before making any entrance, anywhere.

My pool-party example shows you not only the need to make sure you have the right lighting to do your makeup. It also shows that you need to be aware of what you're getting ready for. If I'd been going out to the club, that look could have worked. There's daytime makeup and nighttime makeup, and there's a *big* difference between the two. So be sure to really stop and think about what you're getting dressed for and what kind of impression you want to make, and then take the time and care to prepare accordingly. That way, no matter the occasion, you'll completely own it.

> *A bad bitch always walks into a room feeling like she owns it, so do everything in your power to make sure you look your best.*

Your makeup is more likely to look amazing if you properly prepare the canvas on which you're painting. The better you care for your skin, the more you will glow, no matter how much—or little—makeup you wear. Most dermatologists, aestheticians, and makeup artists will tell you there are three steps to flawless skin: cleanse, tone, moisturize.

Cleansing is all about finding the best product for your skin type—again, do your research, not only by reading magazines and online tips, but also by talking to an aesthetician, or even just a clerk at a beauty supply store, who can help you to assess what your particular skin needs to keep it healthy and glowing. Most products should be used twice a day, in the morning and before bed, and removed with lukewarm water. Beware of hot water, which can overdry your skin. Follow any other special instruc-

tions on the product. When done, pat your face with a clean towel.

Toner is helpful for removing any makeup, dirt, or oil that may have evaded your face wash. But it's important not to strip or overdry your skin by using a toner that's too harsh.

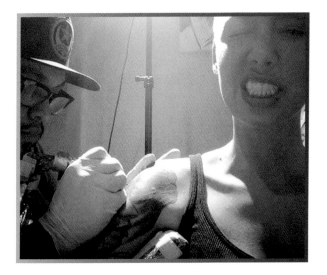

Again, be careful to choose the best product for your skin type and use it as directed. Ideal toners are water-based and pH balanced.

Picking out the right moisturizer for your skin is perhaps the most complicated step in the process, and also the most important. Using the wrong type of moisturizer for your skin type can clog your pores and lead to dull or greasy skin, or even breakouts. But going without moisturizer can cause your skin to become overly dry and produce excess oil to compensate. During the day, it's best to wear an SPF when you're outside, even for short periods, in order to avoid sun damage. Sometimes it can be easier to wear a moisturizer that also contains an SPF, or you may want to choose two separate products because of their individual benefits. On the other hand, when you moisturize before bed, you don't want to use a product with an SPF, so you may want to choose a separate nighttime cream. Again, getting some advice about the best way to protect your skin, depending on your skin type and budget, can always help.

I take care of my skin, and now it takes care of me in return. I don't ever skip a step, no matter how late it is when I get home and even when I'm traveling. They don't call it a skin-care routine for nothing.

No matter how tired you are at night or how rushed you are in the morning, you've got to take the time to do all three steps. I use Clinique because they have a three-part system that works together. That way, I don't have to think about it. For years, I washed my face with Dove soap. And for moisturizer, I used these little containers of raw African shea butter, which I bought from street vendors, warmed up in the microwave before using the cream to drench my entire body—skin, scalp, and face. But then I wanted something even simpler, so I found Clinique, which makes a coordinated system that works well for me. I still use the shea butter on my body, though. And I don't plan to ever do anything more complicated than this. I'm a big believer in keeping it simple. I believe that using too much of too many different products can backfire on you by overwhelming your skin.

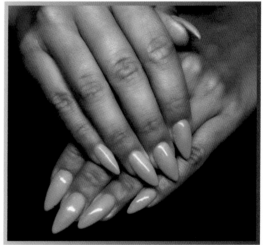

There are a million options out there. Don't use them all at once, but don't be afraid to experiment until you find one or two that really suit your skin. Again, don't miss the chance to ask others for guidance, either. Believe me, if you see a gorgeous woman and you tell her that she has beautiful skin and you want to know her secrets, she is going to be flattered as hell, and she is going to tell you what products she uses, plus all her tips for making everything work.

Being a bad bitch is as much in the details as it is in the grand gestures, and taking care of yourself is the foundation of everything else you do in your life.

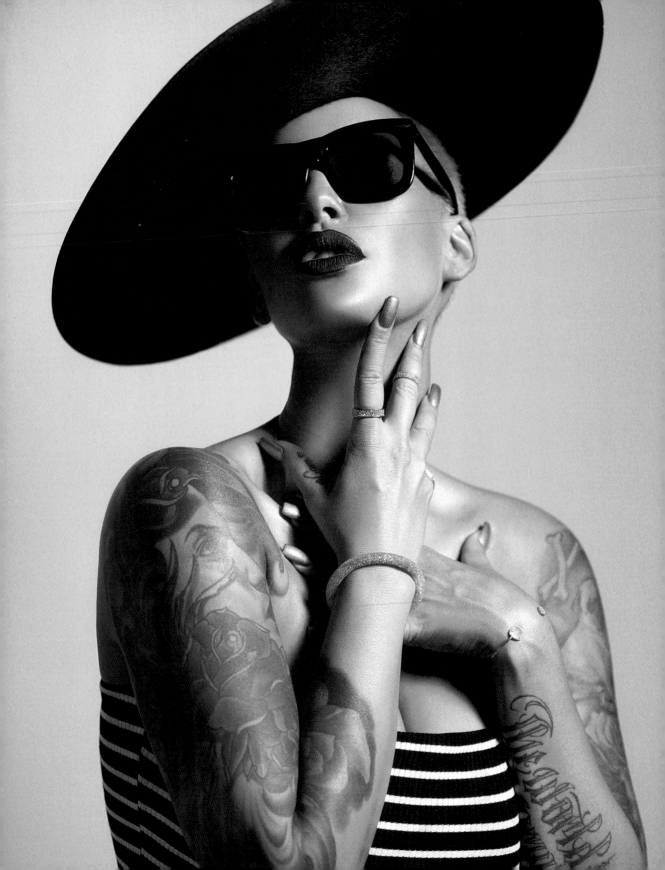

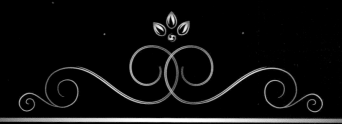

3
FASHION

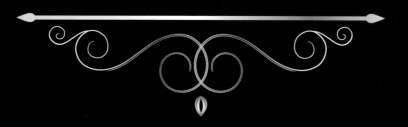

I love fashion, but I don't love the fashion industry. It seems the fashion "experts" and the fashion "insiders" always want to tell everyone what they need to wear this particular season because it's what's in style.

Fuck that. Fashion is not about being a slave to trends. Fashion is self-expression. Fashion is feeling good because you're wearing something on the outside that reveals who you really are on the inside. You should only wear clothes that represent your personality. That's how you can be a trendsetter instead of being trendy. Think about people who have true style, people like my current style icons: Pharrell, Gwen Stefani, and Omahyra Mota. They're all unique individuals who dress like no one else does. They do what they feel and what makes them happy, and because of that, they always look great.

My approach to fashion really depends on the day. Sometimes I feel very androgynous. Sometimes I want to be a girly girl in a flowery dress. It's all about how I feel in the morning. It's all about my mood. But I always take the time to create an impression, whether it's butch or femme or somewhere in between. In a world where people size you up in an instant—in real life and on social media—it has never been more important to be in control of your own look and its impact.

Style comes from the inside, for sure. This goes back to the vision of yourself that you created before you did anything else. There wouldn't be new styles if there weren't innovators to create them. Usually, it's the weirdest, most awkward person who comes up with the coolest stuff. All it took was one person being confident enough to try something new as a form of self-expression.

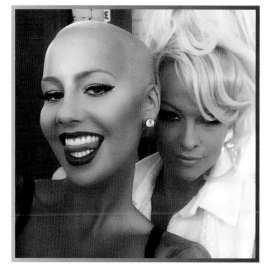

With an original bad bitch: Pamela Anderson

Try your hardest not to live for others. Because when you do that, you're likely to end up unhappy. How could you not if you're trying to please everyone else but not yourself? In reality, you can't control what anyone thinks about you anyhow. All you can control is your own experience of life and your own joy. So you might as well choose to enjoy yourself, right?

Plus, happy people look better, no matter what they're wearing. And you know what? I was *happy* in some of the looks I'm about to tell you about, even if I wouldn't wear them now. That's right, I can't tell you how to find your own bad-bitch style without first telling you how I somehow managed to find mine, without money and with a sometimes disastrous lack of self-consciousness.

I wanted my appearance to please <u>me</u> and no one else.

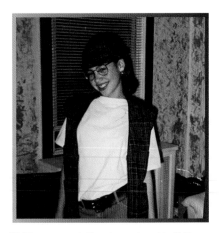

Visiting my cousin Tracy's apartment in Philly when I was twelve. She used to give me all her hand-me-downs, including this hat and vest, which were from the Gap.

I mean, I would wear *anything* if I thought it was cool.

It's not that I set out to look unusual, exactly. I just dressed how I felt. And when I was a kid, I knew I was different. I just was. When I was coming up in South Philly, everyone around me was very hip-hop. I liked hip-hop, but I don't believe in being defined by just one style of music—or just one anything, really. I also loved Pantera, Sinéad O'Connor, Aaliyah, Nirvana, and Guns N' Roses, even though they were a little before my time. And my style borrowed a bit from all of those artists and more. I didn't look like the other kids in my neighborhood. And I didn't want to; I wanted my appearance to please *me* and no one else. Sometimes my look worked, and sometimes it didn't, but I always made an impact, and over time, getting noticed gave me confidence.

INSPIRATION IS ALL AROUND YOU

When I was very young, I loved Cyndi Lauper. Anytime her videos came on, I watched them closely and studied her look. Again, it wasn't like I was going to copy any one particular outfit, item for item, but I wanted to soak up the overall impact of her style and then take it apart and borrow aspects of it for myself. It wasn't just her appearance that I loved, either. I also loved her energy and her fearlessness. And I'd like to think I've incorporated some of all that into the woman I grew up to be.

Over this past winter, I was in the Bahamas for an appearance when a young man came up to me with his phone in his hand. FaceTime was open on the screen. I smiled politely at him, unsure where our conversation was going to lead.

"My mom wants to talk to you on FaceTime," he said.

"OK," I said gamely, even though I had no idea what would happen next.

I looked into the camera, and staring back at me was Cyndi Lauper. I almost screamed. I couldn't believe that *she* wanted to talk to *me*. No matter what else I accomplish in my life, that will always be one of my proudest moments.

Even as a kid, I was always on the lookout for anything that was different, anything that was cool. For instance, when Madonna started wearing suits, I couldn't get enough of how incredible she looked. I thought, *A woman in a suit. That's so hot. One day, I'm going to do that, too.*

I pointed out one of these pictures to a girlfriend.

"You're weird," she said. "Why would you want to put on a suit?"

"Because she's cool," I said.

Mind you, when Madonna struck a pose in a suit in her "Vogue" video, it was 1990. I was six. See, I always knew that when I grew up, I wanted to be a bad bitch.

Express Yourself

When I was young, I didn't believe in matching. It was just too boring. I wanted to wear different socks and different shoes. I mean, like, two *different* shoes, like a red Converse and a yellow one or whatever else struck my fancy that day. I didn't believe in any standards, either. If my mom bought me a really cool pajama set, I would want to wear it to school. And I did. For me, getting dressed every day was a chance to express myself, and I indulged myself fully.

When I was in fifth or sixth grade, my mom took me to Payless for shoes. We were poor as hell, and that was all we could afford. I always went for the most dramatic, awkward-looking shoe, because I thought that was the coolest. I was immediately drawn to these big, bright blue shoes that had two fat elastic straps crisscrossing the top. They were so weird they were kind of cool. But I wasn't sure. They were really strange and almost ugly. *I can't wear these,* I thought. And then, just as quickly, *Nah, I've got to wear them.*

So I wore them to school, and sure enough, all the kids made fun of me. "Your shoes look stupid," they said as I walked down the halls.

To make matters worse, the shoes had big Payless stickers inside them, which I was always trying to hide so people wouldn't tease me for being weird *and* poor. I reached a point, not long after that, where I didn't care what people thought anymore.

But when I was a little kid, I got embarrassed about being broke, even though I knew deep down there was no shame in it, and every other kid in my school and neighborhood was just as broke as me, so there was no point in being embarrassed. And now, I'm so proud of my mom for giving us as much as she did on her single waitress salary.

Well, because we were poor, it wasn't like I had any other shoes to wear, so I kept right on wearing—and loving—my bright blue monstrosities. And the kids kept right on making fun of me. And then, about two weeks in, I noticed a girl in my class was wearing those same Payless shoes everyone had been tearing down just the day before, only hers were red. And the next day, a few people were wearing them in white and black, too, until it seemed like pretty much everyone had a pair of those Payless shoes in one color or another. Clearly, my classmates all knew the shoes came from Payless now, but they weren't about to make fun of me if they were wearing them, too. I didn't say anything or make a big deal of it. I just laughed to myself. But I won't lie; that felt good.

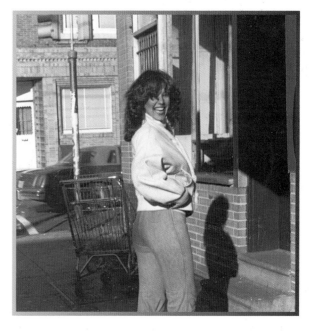

My mom, Dottie, in 1979 at nineteen years old. When my mom sees this photo she says, "I didn't know my own beauty."

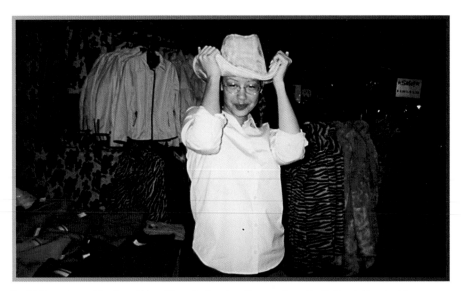

In eighth grade, my friends and I loved to go to the store Guacamole on South Street. They had the coolest clothes.

I've always thought people looked best rocking their own fabulous, unique style, but it was pretty cool to suddenly be a trendsetter. Especially because I had no money to spend on clothes, and so I was always trying to make my look out of whatever I could get.

Before I shaved my head and came into my own, boys never liked me. I dressed and acted so differently from all the other girls. When I'd go knock for my friends, especially in grade school, their parents would say stuff like "The weird girl from down the street is at the door for you." I used to have stuff like that happen to me all the time. But instead of going home and changing, I pushed back.

"I want to wear it," I would say. "Mind your own business."

And I'd even rock my "weird" outfit the next day in front of the same people, and then again later that week, and the next week, until I wore them down.

Even though I didn't fit in with the rest of the girls in South Philly, it got to where I actually liked the attention I received for being different. And then, finally, in around ninth grade, people stopped making fun of me. I guess it had reached the point where everyone knew to expect the unexpected from me. Whereas they used to freak out and say, *"What are you wearing?"* now they'd just say, "Oh, that's Amber. That's nothing shocking. That's not even anything new. That's just her." Eventually, however, the way I wanted to look became normal, and not just to me. It had caught on. But you know what? Even if the people in my neighborhood had never come around to my way of thinking, I would have kept dressing the way I did anyhow.

But even if I had to stand alone, I would, because that's who I am, and I'm proud of it.

Sure, in the moment, getting teased sucked. It didn't feel good at all. But looking back, I'm actually glad it happened that way. Sticking to my vision of the world—from my dream to my look—no matter what anyone said about it actually gave me confidence. And it's that sense of myself, and that self-assurance, that got me where I am today and keeps me moving forward, no matter what kinds of setbacks I might face or what kinds of haters I might encounter. I mostly don't even hear the negative comments anymore, because I got so used to disregarding them all those years ago. And so I'm not afraid to come out against slut-shaming or any other bullshit where people try to tell anyone how to dress or who to be.

No one knows me better than I know myself, and no one knows you better than you know yourself. So let's stand together for our right to be individuals. I've got your back, and I know you've got mine. But even if I had to stand alone, I would, because that's who I am, and I'm proud of it.

WEAR WHAT MAKES YOU FEEL GOOD

A little later, in the late '90s, there was this neighborhood in Philly called South Street that was really popping. That's where most of the city's vintage boutiques and punk-rock record stores were, and you'd see people walking down the street with different-colored hair or Mohawks or ripped-up jeans, long before any of that was cool anywhere else in Philly. I loved it. I couldn't get enough. Seeing all that individuality and creativity made me feel free to try out all the different crazy looks I was starting to come up with in my own head. Soon enough, I was known as one of the South Street kids, because—at least by the hip-hop standards of my neighborhood—everyone on South Street was weird, and I was weird, too.

I did have one friend, Donna, who was also into experimenting with fashion, and she gave me all her cool hand-me-down clothes. She also took me to the best thrift stores in Philly. I grew up poor, so I always went to secondhand stores and tried to find the best gems I could. I was relentless. I would pore over racks and racks of clothes until I uncovered a piece that was just what I'd been looking for—not a particular look I'd thought I'd wanted but a special piece nonetheless. I found inspiration in the fabric or cut or pattern, anything that made me stand out. And, even more important, I made it fit with the vision I had of myself, which was fabulous and glam and worlds away from the streets of Philly or the Goodwill or the Dollar Store.

Even though I never could have told you what I was looking for ahead of time, I always knew it when I saw it. My favorite thrift-store find from back then was a yellow dress with black polka dots. It kind of looked like the outfit a small-town waitress would wear, but

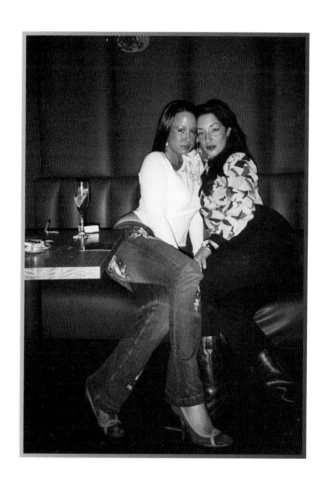

At my twenty-second birthday party with one of my best friends, Donna, who always took me thrift store shopping. (By the way, I'm wearing a wig in this picture.)

that's what made it dope. It was so cute, and it became my favorite dress; I wore it all the time. That was the best piece I ever found at a secondhand store, for sure.

I found my other favorite look from back then when I was about fourteen years old. This was in '97 or '98. I started working at a store on South Street called Unica. We got in a complete Guess outfit made out of a special kind of treated denim that was almost shiny. It had a matching jacket and pants, and each piece cost $120. Back then, that was a lot of money, especially for me. But I had to have it. So I put it on layaway, and I kept it in my mind: *I am going to get that outfit. I am going to get that outfit.* Finally, I'd saved up enough money and brought it home. I wore it *every single day.* I was obsessed.

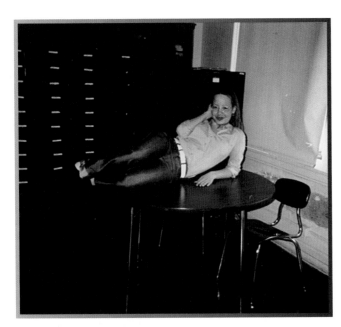

Modeling the shiny Guess jeans I saved up to buy while working at Unica. I loved that outfit!

Wear what makes you feel good, and never be afraid to express yourself through your style, even if it varies from day to day. I was never just the sexy girl, although I definitely liked to dress that way sometimes. I also rocked menswear and was comfortable dressing androgynously. There was a moment in my fashion evolution when I wore Dickies shorts with Chucks and little cutoff tank tops, à la Gwen Stefani. I shopped at Hot Topic and dressed like a punk rocker sometimes, too. What I wore depended on the day and my mood and what was going on in my life.

Whatever I was wearing, I felt good because it came from me, and that made me feel like I looked good, which made all the difference in how I saw myself.

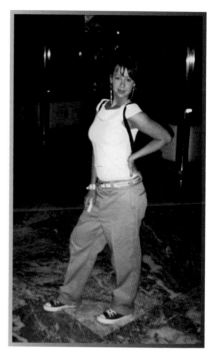

At a casino when I was twenty-one and going through my Dickie's phase.

BE COMFORTABLE IN YOUR OWN SKIN

To be honest, I've always been very confident with my body, and I never felt ashamed of having curves or of wanting to flaunt them. Sure, it was sometimes hard coming into my own, but the older I got, the more powerful I felt. And from the time I was a teenager, I never let anyone make me feel less than perfect, inside and out. Not even close. I never let anyone control me, either. Harnessing my own power was a conscious choice, and I have chosen to stick with it ever since.

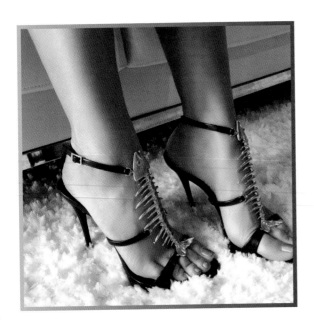

Before I fully took control of my inner bad bitch, my mom used to try to steer me in her direction and toward her vision when I started doing my own thing as a teenager. Here is a story about how well that went for her. In high school, I'd put on sweatpants and a sweatshirt and head out the door to hang with my friends, like nothing was up. But I was *really* wearing little booty shorts and a tank top underneath, and as soon as I got out of view of our apartment, I'd strip down to my sexy outfit and hang out with my friends on the corner, all of us dressed exactly the same, like we were at the beach and not on the block.

One day, a car pulled up, and the passenger window rolled down. There was my stepdad driving, my mom riding shotgun, and she was pissed.

"Get your fucking ass in the car right now," she said. "I'm cutting up those shorts when we get home."

I gave her a look that said, *Go ahead and make me,* but I knew better than to disobey her when she was in *that* mood.

As soon as we got home, she made me go change. When she was in a state like this, I knew better than to try to argue with her, so I put on some baggy sweats and came out of the bathroom carrying my other clothes. My mom was standing in the living room with a pair of scissors in her hand.

"Give them to me," she said.

I handed them over, glaring at her as she started cutting my booty shorts into shreds and then did the same thing to my tank top.

"Mom, I hate you! Why are you doing this?" I yelled at her.

At that age, I didn't understand that she was trying to make sure I had the chance to live all my dreams, so I mouthed off. But of course, now that I'm older, I can see my mom's point, and I'm grateful she helped me to reach my potential.

Even when she was yanking me off the street, worried about my choices, she never said a negative word to me about who I was. She was used to my very free spirit. She knew I was different, and she loved and accepted me anyway. She was trying to protect me and keep me from getting tangled up the way a lot of other girls in our neighborhood did. So many girls I came up with got attention from the wrong guys and ended up with babies in high school or drug problems or both. Monique had four kids, all by the same guy, but he was in and out of prison for fifteen years, and she wound up with a drug problem, sometimes having to live in a shelter. My mom wasn't about to let me go down like that, because she wanted me to have every opportunity in the world to create my own life for myself before I became a mom. So she was mad at my outfit, not mad at me.

Choosing our own clothes is one of the first independent decisions we make as young women.

Obviously, I was a teenager at that time, and I didn't have much perspective on life. I didn't understand how young I truly was. It wasn't that I wanted to disrespect my mom or rebel or anything like that. I just felt she didn't understand why it was so important for me to choose what to wear. She didn't understand who I was becoming. As teenagers, choosing our own clothes is one of the first independent decisions we make as young women. And at that moment, dressing in booty shorts was a choice I was making and no one else. That's what was important to me.

Now, I know that not everyone will interpret my booty shorts as a form of self-empowerment. But truly, many women dress sexy in order to feel sexy on the inside, rather than for a guy, and that's awesome. That's what being a bad bitch is all about—living life and making choices for yourself and not for anybody else. Sure, it's nice when there's a positive outcome. It's flattering when a cool guy finds you sexy. But that's not the end-all-be-all. Seriously, we are *way* better than that. We run our own shit, for ourselves.

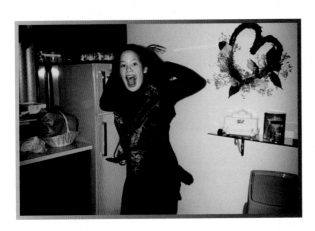

Christmas Eve at my Poppy's house when I was eight or nine. I loved that brown velvet outfit.

Be an Original

Now all of this seems funny. I feel grateful that I had the confidence to be an original. When I read interviews with people who are famous and artsy and really cool—musicians, fashion designers, artists—so many of them faced the same obstacles I did growing up. When I was a kid, though, I thought I was alone in my out-there fashion choices because they made me the black sheep in my family and in my neighborhood.

I wouldn't say it bothered me, exactly. But I never understood why people couldn't accept me for who I was. To them, they were just making fun of my clothes because they looked different. But to me, my clothes let me express my individuality, and so it was like if they had a problem with my clothes, they had a problem with me. So that was hard for me. Over time, though, my attitude became, *if someone doesn't understand or accept who you are, fuck them.* That attitude gave me a really clear sense of who I was and what was important to me early on.

Although I'm not going to tell you *what* to wear, I am going to offer this piece of advice on what *not* to wear:

Shoes that don't fit you: Seriously, wear your shoe size. That's fashion rule number one. Your feet will thank you, and you'll walk with greater ease, which will translate into greater presence and poise.

The wrong shoes for the occasion: There are walking heels, and then

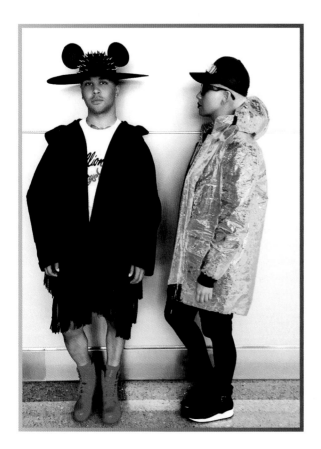

there are sit-at-the-bar-and-look-cute heels, for when all you do is go from your car to the bar and then back to the car. I have shoes like that. I wouldn't dare walk down Hollywood Boulevard in them, because they fucking hurt, and I would look crazy. Or I would wind up taking them off and walking barefoot, and then I'd *really* look crazy. So be sure you dress appropriately for whatever you're about to do.

A dress you can't move in: When you try on a dress at the

store, bend over. Sit down. Know exactly what you're going to do when you wear that dress, and make sure it fits you in all different scenarios.

The wrong size bra: Believe it or not, most women have no idea what bra size they truly are. So even if you *think* you know, get measured. Have you ever worn a bra that slips down when you bend over? All of us have, and it means you need to get fitted ASAP. Wearing a bra that's too small is not only bad for you (think back pain and bad posture), but it's also extremely unflattering. Boost your self-esteem by getting fitted for a proper bra that will not only provide the support you need but also transform your look in ways you can't even imagine until you see it.

Clothes that don't work with your shape: We've all seen girls—heavier or skinnier—wearing clothes that just aren't flattering to their bodies, and it's clear they feel self-conscious, and that's not a good look. If you're not feeling good in something, don't pretend in order to follow a trend. Be honest with yourself.

SHAME-FREE ZONE

Women shouldn't be ashamed of their size, no matter how big or small they are. There's nothing sexier than a woman owning her body. And a huge part of this is embracing your curves if you've got them, while also making use of all the tools you have to enhance your assets. So yes, I believe in Spanx.

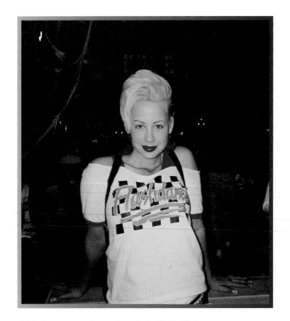

A Marilyn moment, age twenty, in Philly. This was definitely when I was all about Gwen Stefani, too.

It is one of the best undergarments in the world; it creates clean lines and streamlines every woman's figure. Spanx takes the best of you and makes it better, which can only boost your confidence. And Spanx is for skinny girls, too. Women of every size and shape should feel entitled to wear the shortest, tightest, sexiest clothes they want without anyone saying anything to them. So if you feel good in a micromini without Spanx, go for it. Your attitude is the most important part of any outfit, and I trust you to decide what looks good on you.

Don't get confused, though. If you're having a date night and you think things might get a little frisky, do not wear Spanx. There's nothing worse in the heat of the moment than having to wriggle out of something super-tight, so plan ahead.

Curvy or skinny, tall or short, we all look better with smooth lines under our clothes, and that's why properly fitted bras and Spanx are our best friends. There's nothing more confidence-shattering than items that don't fit right, and undergarments are the foundation of everything else. If you have the power to make yourself look and feel better, why not use it as your secret weapon?

If you can rock a look with confidence, you can get away with pretty much anything. It's most important for you to feel comfortable with what you have on. That's really the only rule. Feel good in your clothes, whatever they are, and you'll always look amazing.

Fantasies Are Meant to Feel Good

Now that you've heard my style story and tips it's time to figure out your look. So where should you begin? A great way to get inspired and start dreaming is to look backward at some of the gorgeous and fabulous ladies and gents who came before us. I've always been obsessed with studying pictures and videos of my people—the ones who rock my favorite looks and attitudes—and taking cues from them. When I was coming up, my fashion icons were Grace Jones, Madonna, Slash, Sinéad O'Connor, Aaliyah, Gwen Stefani, and Omahyra Mota. I've still been known to keep an eye on what Gwen and Omahyra are up to, even now that I've mastered the fundamentals of what works for my look and what doesn't. I'm always excited to see what others are wearing and draw fresh inspiration from them.

When you see a dope look online or in a magazine, don't think that's just for *them* because they're rich or famous or thin or any other qualifiers you can use to put yourself down if you're not careful. Instead, picture yourself in that look. Think about how it would feel, or what you might do differently for your particular size, style, and comfort zone. Have fun. Fantasies are meant to feel good, you know?

Once you've got the image in your mind, think about how to make it work for you. I'm not talking about recreating the exact look of some famous person and walking around like some cookie-cutter version of her. Dare to mix it up. Get fresh. Take one piece of one look and combine it with something else. Maybe the heels are too high—or not high enough. Maybe you feel sexier in tight skirts, or maybe hip-hugging jeans are your thing. If you feel good, you'll look good.

Once you envision yourself a certain way, then do it, no matter what. If you see yourself looking like a Bohemian hippie type of chick, but all your friends are into tight dresses and high heels, go against the grain. It's only

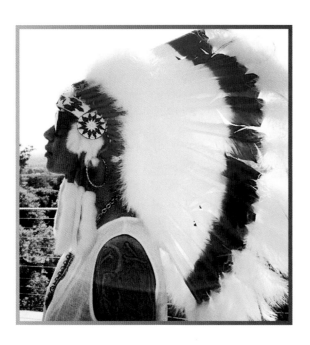

going to earn you more attention. When you feel comfortable with who you are, your poise will shine through.

I hope you won't be afraid to stand out. You could follow the hot new styles you see in every magazine and then show up to a party only to find someone else wearing the same thing. Or you could wear your favorite silk pajamas or your favorite old concert T-shirt or your one-of-a-kind yellow polka-dot vintage dress and be the hottest, most original woman there. Always be true to yourself, and you'll look your best.

By now, I hope you're getting the picture that you can be a bad bitch in a sweat suit, as long as you're owning it. While I do have some practical advice here in these pages, being a bad bitch isn't really about following a how-to book; it means doing whatever it takes to fully own your own power.

Sure, plenty of fashion magazines will tell you exactly how to dress, what's hot and what's not. Articles like that can be useful in small doses. Honestly, though, I'm so over that shit. I'm over magazines that tell women how they should look and, in turn, tell women that they aren't all that if they don't look a certain way. I think it's a large part of why girls have become so self-conscious and insecure. Just because a woman can't rock a pair of hipless tuxedo pants or, conversely, fill out a full-busted corset, doesn't mean she's less than beautiful. If you can't achieve a certain look exactly as it's represented in the glossies, don't think, *That's not for me. I can't be pretty. I can't be sexy. I don't have the money. I don't have the eye for it. I don't have the body. I don't have the beauty.*

Fuck that. No more.

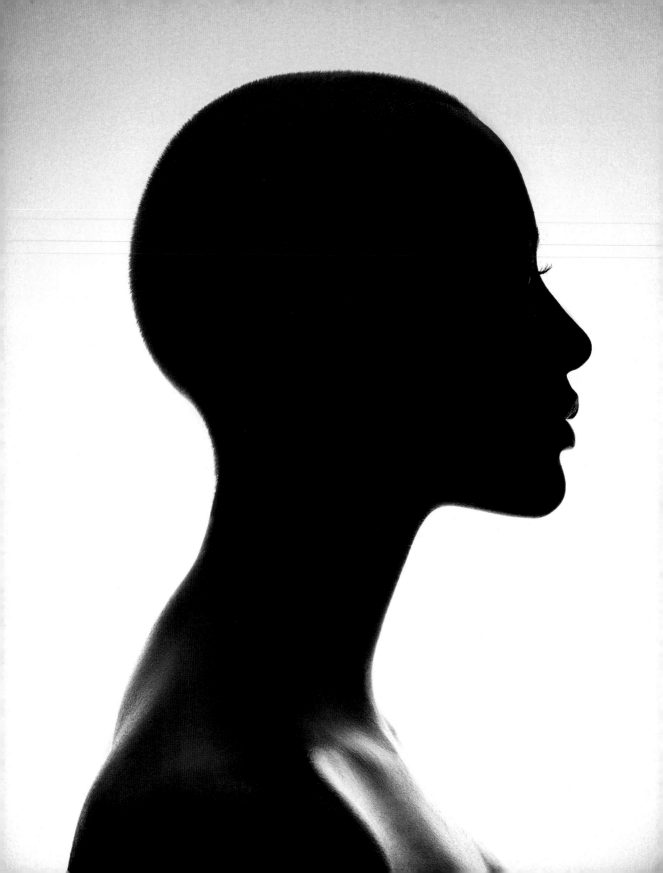

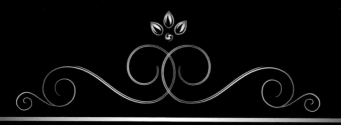

4

INNER STRENGTH

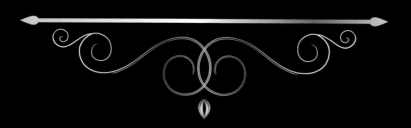

Now that we've worked on your vision and learned a few things about using beauty and fashion to bring your best self to life, we're ready to take the most important step of all: it's time to give this bitch a soul. In order to do that, you have to tap into your inner strength. You might grow strong because of the obstacles life places in your path, or from your own determination. Either way, it'll give you the power you need to create your best self and help you feel confident, which is the bad bitch way.

SOMETIMES YOU HAVE TO FIGHT

The thing is, I didn't have a choice but to learn how to be strong and stand up for myself. Where I grew up, it was a matter of survival. When I was fourteen, I hadn't had sex yet, which was unusual for a girl in my neighborhood. But like most teenage girls, I was getting into boys. I'd heard that this girl, Paula, from the next neighborhood over had sex with the boy I liked. That made me jealous, so I ran my mouth.

"That Paula, she's such a fucking ho," I said to a friend of mine.

See, at that young age, I didn't know any better than to slut-shame a girl, just because I was mad she got the guy I liked. These days, I'm determined to speak out against slut-shaming and teach girls coming up not to slut-shame each other or let anyone do it

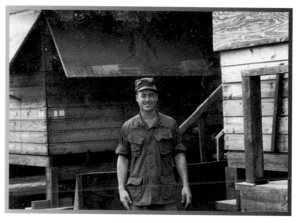

My dad, Michael, when he was stationed in Fort Dix, New Jersey. He taught me a lot about how to stand up for myself.

to them, but I had to learn that lesson the hard way. As I was about to find out, a friend told Paula what I'd said. A few days later, I was with another friend, Tiffany, on our way home from Jason Douglas Dancing School, when Paula jumped out of a car with her boyfriend, Steve, her best friend, Jen, and her aunt.

When I saw Steve, my heart sank. He wasn't the guy I liked who Paula had supposedly been with. In fact, he tortured me, and he'd always been the person in my neighborhood who bullied me worse than anyone else. Just the week before, he'd made me cry by calling me the meanest names imaginable. He was incredibly cruel and totally relentless, and I knew today would be no different. They were there to fight me, and I had no choice but to stand my ground. In a neighborhood like that, you had to fight, because if you didn't, you would never live it down, and you'd get beat up every single day.

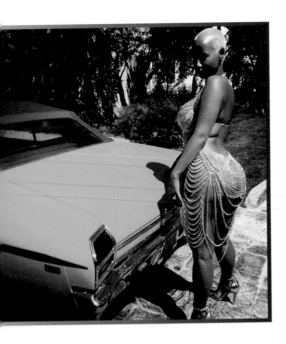

Paula rolled up on me, glaring. "Yo, bitch," she said. "I hear you called me a ho."

I didn't hesitate for a minute, because I knew I couldn't. I was already pulling my hair into a ponytail and wrapping it up so she couldn't grab it and use it against me. Tiffany was no longer anywhere to be seen. I was on my own. "Well, I can't help what you are," I said.

She threw the first punch at me. And then I let her have it.

And so now Steve got involved. "You going to let Amber beat your ass like that?" he taunted her. "You better get up and teach her a lesson."

I wasn't afraid now. Instead, I thought, *OK, bitch, round two. That's cool.*

Round two started, and again I was getting the better of her. Finally, her friend Jen jumped in and got me down on the sidewalk. Jen started pulling my hair and kicking me. Steve jumped in and kicked me in my ribs, and then Paula's aunt started pulling my hair, too. They didn't stop until they'd beaten the crap out of me.

Finally, they left me on the ground and sped off in their car.

I was two blocks away from home, and I was afraid they were going to come back for me. I got myself up and, hurt as I was, started running.

Our apartment was on the third floor, and normally I yelled up for my mom to throw down the key for me. This time, as I got to the corner of our block, I started shouting, "Mom! Mom! Come outside right now! They just jumped me!"

My mom ran downstairs. When she reached the street, she was carrying the white cane that belonged to our neighbor on the second floor, who was legally blind and usually left her cane just inside the front door of our building. I told my mom what happened, and she was furious that a grown woman had been beating on her fourteen-year-old daughter, so she went after them.

Just then, they pulled down my block, looking for me. The aunt was driving, and my mom waved them over.

"Bitch, get the fuck out of the car right now," my mom said. "You put your fucking hands on my daughter?"

They took one look at how pissed my mom was, and they sped off. Well, everyone in my neighborhood and Paula's neighborhood heard that I'd beaten her up in the first and second rounds and that she'd been reduced to having a whole group of people jump in and beat me up for her. Nobody fucked with me after that.

I didn't enjoy my victory for long, though. Maybe a month or two later, it came out that Paula had cancer. All the kids in my neighborhood could be really cruel, and they started teasing me about this.

"Amber gave Paula cancer," they said.

I was so naive that I believed them, and that was really heavy on me. I actually went home from school one day and talked to my mom about it. "Mom, could I have really given her cancer?"

"No, baby, you had a fight," she said. "That's all. You didn't give her no cancer."

Even when I was old enough to know that my mom was right, I still felt bad for Paula. I had compassion for her and her suffering, and I didn't like thinking about how we'd fought over something so stupid. I never wanted to fight again, and I made a point not to trash-talk anyone, especially when I was just jealous or angry.

I'm actually glad for that fight, though, because it allowed me to learn how strong I am. I still draw on that confidence in my ability to handle myself when I need to in business—well, in all areas of my life. Sometimes you've got to take care of a situation, even if you're scared or you don't want to deal with it.

I may have learned my lesson from that early fight, but it still felt good many years later, when I was back visiting Philly from Hollywood and ran into Steve. By this point, my modeling career had taken off, and I was doing well for myself. Steve, on the other hand, was clearly a junkie. He was emaciated and had pockmarks all over. Even so, he had the balls to try to take me home. I couldn't believe it. He had made my life hell for years. He had beaten me up. And now he was hitting on me?

"You know who I am, right?" I said.

"Yeah, yeah, yeah, Amber, we grew up together, baby," he said. "I mean, I've known you since we were kids."

"You don't even know the trauma you created in my life when I was a kid," I said. "And you have the audacity to try to come at me right now? No fucking way, dude. Go fuck yourself."

It felt incredible. I got to have the moment we'd all like to have with our childhood bullies. It was fucking sweet.

You'll have your moment someday, too, even if it doesn't come in quite that form. No matter what stage of life you're at right now, keep reminding yourself that it will get better. Just keep being your bad bitch self, and it will all work out the way it's supposed to in the end, with you ruling your own life on your own terms and no thought for any of the haters. All of the hard stuff that happens along the way sucks at the time, I know, but the good news is that it only makes you stronger.

ACT CONFIDENT, AND PEOPLE WON'T KNOW ANY BETTER

I think half the time we get criticized, it's because we're giving off vibes that we're looking for approval or even just acceptance. People can smell weakness, and it doesn't bring out the best in everyone. But radiate power and self-acceptance, and that sends a whole different message. Not only does it give you the advantage in your dealings with others, but it also will draw them to you. Others will see you feeling good about yourself, and they'll want some of that for themselves, too.

People can smell weakness, and it doesn't bring out the best in everyone. But radiate power and self-acceptance, and that sends a whole different message.

It's not always an easy thing to do, especially on tough days, which I'm well acquainted with. Sometimes all you've got is your willpower. No matter how down and out you might feel, you've got to get yourself up in the morning. Get into the shower, get dressed, do your makeup so you feel pretty, and then get out of the house. This may sound like a bullshit way of dealing with what might be some pretty dark days in your life. But I've had days as dark as anyone else, if not darker, and I know that how you approach them really helps.

When I have hard days, I do anything and everything to stay busy. That way, at the end of the night, I'm so exhausted that I can sleep instead of staying up and worrying. I don't really sleep much; I never have. So I have to wear myself out. There have been days when I make sure I'm doing something every second—not that this is difficult these days; being a mom keeps me busy in the most rewarding way possible. There's nothing better in the world than having the first thing I hear be my son's sweet little voice: "Mommy, I want orange juice." After that, it's not hard for me to get out of bed with a smile on my face. But if I just lie in bed or let myself sit around watching TV, I will fall into a pit.

I started experiencing depression and anxiety when I was twelve years old. Depression definitely runs in my family, so maybe it was hereditary. Or maybe it's just how I'm wired. I also had my first panic attack at age twelve. Not that I knew what it was at the time. All of a sudden, my peripheral vision started to vanish. Everything I looked at seemed a little off. I did what I always did when I had a problem: I went to my mom.

"Mommy, I think I need a new prescription for my glasses, because I can't see right," I said. "There's something wrong."

My mom took me to the doctor. They couldn't find anything wrong with me, but I started having this feeling frequently, like everything was suddenly animated and I was in a different

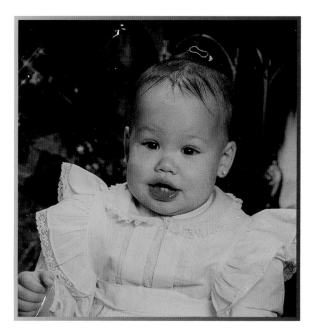

This is my mom's favorite picture. It was taken when I was around a year old. When she looks at it now, she says I have Bash's eyes.

world. I learned to start talking myself down: *Amber, this is real life. You're not in a movie right now. Everything is fine. Just calm down. This is no big deal.*

Finally, with a little practice, I got to where I could manage my anxiety. And I leaned some tricks for minimizing it. I eventually went to a doctor who diagnosed me with panic attacks and gave me medication for moments when I was having severe anxiety. Scientists understand how the brain works so much better than they did when I was a kid, and just knowing what's going on with me has helped a lot.

You've got to get back out there in order to get back on top.

If you're feeling anything like this, I definitely recommend that you go to a doctor. Like me, if you've been living with a problem like this for years, you might be amazed by how much better you can feel. I know I have been.

Also, I don't drink coffee, and I try to stay away from caffeinated sodas, even though with my schedule, I sometimes really need that boost. But I'm always very mindful of how much caffeine I have, because I know it can trigger my anxiety.

For the average bad day, I try to surround myself with the pick-me-ups that can easily turn my mood around. That's definitely my son; his smile and his voice are enough to cheer me up instantly. Loud music helps to pep me up, too. Anything really upbeat, anything I can dance to, improves my mood. When I'm really down, I'll let myself listen to songs about heartbreak or betrayal or anger—whatever it is I'm feeling—and I'll crank them, and I'll cry and sing along at the top of my voice, getting everything out. But then I'll cut myself off. No R&B, no sad love songs, nothing that's going to make me cry. It's one thing to grieve something for a few days, maybe a week, but after that, you're not doing yourself any favors. You've got to get back out there in order to get back on top.

I also have a rule that I stay off social media when I'm feeling bad; if you're sad or having anxiety, social media is not the place to make you feel better. There's so much extreme negativity out there. You don't want to feel even worse because you see people being mean to others—or being mean to you—

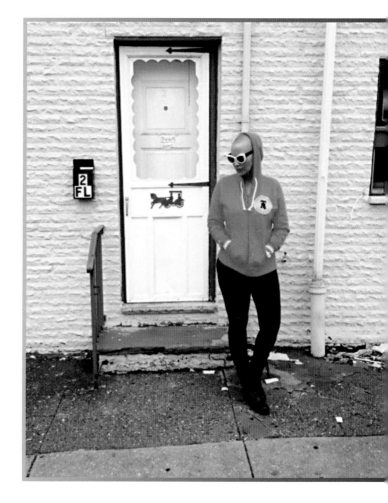

Visiting the apartment I grew up in. I am forever humbled by my life—I always stay strong cause I'm a down home South Philly girl at heart.

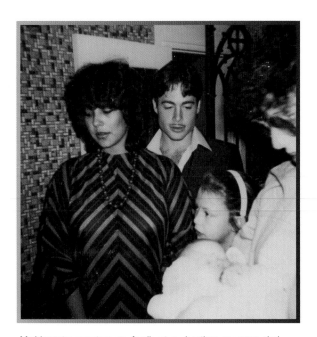

My biggest supporters, my family, at my baptism: my mom; dad; and baby me, being held by my dad's sister, my aunt Beverly (my godmother); and my cousin Tracy, who got too close to the candle during the ceremony. When her hair caught fire, the adults had to use holy water to put it out. Never a dull moment!

and you don't want to laugh at how other people are getting put down, because that urge people have to make themselves feel better by making fun of other people is poison. You might think it feels good in the moment, but it's empty satisfaction, like how junk food is empty calories. You don't want to be that person. You also don't want to be the person who airs out all your personal information on social media. I know I've made that mistake before. I'm teaching you what I've learned the hard way.

If you're feeling down, reach out to close friends and family members. You might feel like you're alone, but you're not. And being reminded that there are people who care about you can help so much. I know it helps me. I really hope you've got someone in your life you can talk to, but if you don't, there are resources out there. Doctors, counselors, hotlines. Seriously, you matter too much not to take care of yourself and do everything you can to turn things around.

BELIEVE IN YOURSELF
AND OTHERS WILL, TOO

I can't stress enough how much my mom helped me in the self-esteem department. I was her only child, so I got all of her attention and praise, and there was a lot of it. Everything I did was such a big deal. Every time I drew a picture, she told me it was beautiful and hung it on the fridge. Every day when I got ready for school, she told me I was amazing. She really made me believe it. Anytime people criticized me or made fun of me, I weighed what they were saying against the much more substantial evidence I had in my life: *My mom says I'm the shit, so I'm the shit.*

Even though I felt confident enough to be myself, brushing off what other people said, it definitely got to me sometimes (after all, sometimes negativity gets to all of us). I remember coming home from school and sitting down with my mom in the living room of our apartment.

"They think I'm so weird, Mom," I said. "What's wrong with me?"

And mind you, looking back, I appeared insane to the average person. But my mom just beamed at me.

"Amber, you are amazing," she said. "You are beautiful."

How lucky was I to have that kind of support in my life? I know not everyone has the good fortune to grow up with a mom like mine. But you can create the same kind of positive reinforcement for yourself. It's all a matter of how you talk to yourself inside your head. If you're fixating on your flaws and tearing yourself down in the mirror, that negativity is going to be reflected on the outside. But if you can create a little voice inside your head that's as supportive and loving as my mom's—a little voice that tells you you're incredible every day, no matter what—you will glow from the inside out, and it will make all the difference in how people see you and treat you. I know it's not always easy to turn around the way you think, but like everything else, it can be done with a little mindfulness and a lot of practice.

To be a bad bitch, you need self-confidence, just like you need an inspired, polished look that is completely and totally you. So consider this an equally important—if not even more important—part of your homework. Just like you practice putting on your makeup every day until you master all the techniques, practice talking to yourself in a new, more positive way. If it takes a while to turn around the years of negativity you might have received

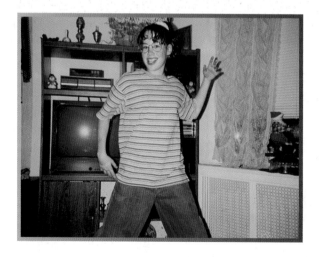

from your family or the kids at school, that's OK. The things in life that are most worth doing often take a little time.

Even then I danced with confidence! This is me at my mom's friend's house, showing them my cool moves.

It All Comes from You

I know it's not so easy to see the world positively, especially if your family never boosted you up, supported you, complimented you, or advocated for your individuality. Even worse, many parents fill their kids up with negativity or abuse. I truly hope that has never happened to you. But if it has, you can turn it around. You can conquer any bad experiences from your past. You really can. Because it all comes from within; it all comes from you. Make a commitment to take the smallest steps every day. Seriously, start by getting up every morning, doing your makeup, and making the choice to look your most beautiful, even if you're just in the house. It's a subtle but powerful reminder that you're not living for anyone but yourself, and all the pleasure and power and joy in life starts and ends with you. Every single day. If you get used to making a commitment to yourself and taking care of yourself, regardless of anything else, it will build your confidence.

Another step you can take is to wear a sexy matching bra-and-panties set, even on a normal Saturday afternoon when you're just lazing around the house. When you wear sweet lingerie under your clothes, it makes you feel sexier, and that confidence radiates outward so you look beautiful to everyone—most important, to yourself. It's also a reminder that your sex appeal or beauty isn't defined by anyone else. You're not wearing that set for anyone else. You are your own audience, your own VIP, and this will reinforce your sense of power. You do you for you.

If you can completely let go of any negativity you hear from others, whether it's on social media or out in the world, and instead embrace the person you are, you'll become the baddest (and happiest) girl there is.

I get a ton of negativity thrown my way every day, and I don't let it affect who I am or how I live. I've never wasted any time caring what people thought of me, and that's definitely made it a lot easier for me to live such a public lifestyle. It's made it easier for me just to be human and have a heightened sense of empathy, too.

It's still a challenge for me to deal with negativity, though, especially when I feel like I'm being attacked. Not long ago, people claimed I'd been Photoshopping the pictures I post on social media. And then the tabloids started posting all of the unflattering pictures of me they could find

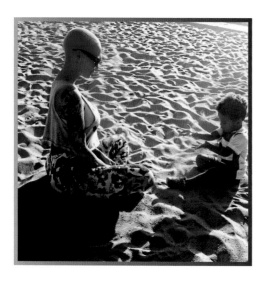

and writing mean things about how ugly I am and how much cellulite I have. Yes, I do have cellulite, actually, and I've never tried to deny it. And, yes, the paparazzi takes unflattering pictues of me all the time, and that's just something I have to deal with in this lifestyle.

I could have easily let all of that negativity get me down, especially because the accusations weren't true. The photo that was supposedly retouched wasn't. I just know how to take a picture from the right angle to make it look as flattering as possible. And yes, I put a sunny filter on it. But that was it.

This kind of thing happens to people who aren't celebrities, too. Think of all the times one of your friends has posted a picture on social media where she looks gorgeous, and you're somewhere in the background with your side boob popping out, looking crazy. Anyone who's caught from a bad angle can take an extremely unflattering picture.

You have to live with integrity, self-assurance, and honesty, no matter what.

Have you ever seen that segment Jimmy Kimmel does on his show where he has celebrities read the mean Tweets about them? It's funny. It's meant to show that Internet hate is laughable and dismissible. The only problem: that's easier said than done. Because those are real people, just like you and me, and those are real things other people have written about them. I know how it feels. So many of us, famous or not, get Tweets like that all the time:

You're fuckin' ugly.

You're bald.

That's why your husband left you, because you're a fuckin' whore.

People write extremely mean things, sometimes targeting really difficult moments in my life. Take the stories from earlier this year, for instance, saying that I'm a bad mom, my house is disgusting, and my

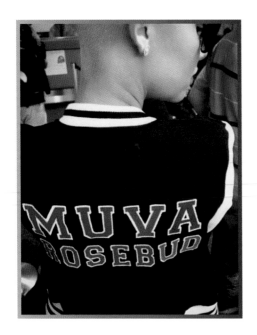

son steps in dog shit *inside* our house. That was extremely painful for me. My son and his health and well-being come before anything else in my life. And to have anyone suggest otherwise made me furious.

Think about it. If it was true, I'd have Child Protective Services coming in and taking my kid away. Of course, it wasn't an accurate story, and the vultures eventually moved on, and it all blew over. But when that was all anyone was talking about, I had to decide not to let it get to me. I had to remind myself that I'm a good mom, and my son knows it, and the people close to me do, too. Because living this very public lifestyle that I do, if I let that kind of stuff get to me, I'd go crazy. And no matter what gets said about me or how untrue it is, I can't comment on it; if I do, I'm just feeding the monster. So no matter how painful it is to imagine people thinking the worst things about my mothering, I have to let it go.

I definitely got trained in not letting negativity get to me, what with all the teasing I endured as I kid. I know a lot of women haven't figured it out yet, though. Many women take the word *sensitive* to the extreme; it becomes important for *everyone* to like them. There's nothing wrong with that, except for the fact that it's impossible. There is no way that every single person you encounter will think the world of you. Part of being a bad bitch is realizing that you have to live with integrity, self-assurance, and honesty, no matter what, and not everyone's going to like it. But the good news is that when you really love yourself, you will care less about what others think and say. That's power.

WHAT OTHER PEOPLE THINK ABOUT YOU IS NONE OF YOUR CONCERN

You've got to focus on you. It's the only way to be happy, and it will plant the seeds of self-esteem within you that will fully bloom over time. Have you ever seen a girl on a dance floor who isn't very attractive but truly does not give a fuck what anybody says about her, and she is just killing it and having the most fun in the whole club, and all the guys *love* her? Maybe she doesn't look like what they typically hold up as their definition of a hot girl, but right there in that moment, she's redefining their perceptions and expanding their idea of what's gorgeous and sexy and desirable. It's because she has the confidence to go out there and not care about how she looks or the impact she's having. She's

A bad bitch doesn't worry or try to make a certain impression. She's too busy living.

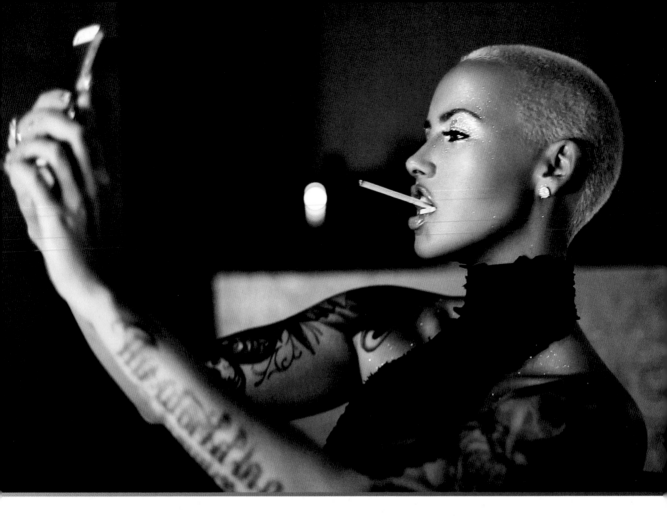

so confident that the guys look past any flaws she might have, even if she wouldn't have been the first girl they picked otherwise. To me, that example is very important, because it's a perfect representation of a bad bitch. I used to see this all the time, especially when I was younger and was out at the clubs more. I observed it. And I learned from it. This is what I came to know: fearlessness is what's attractive to most people, rather than being a size two or having the latest purse or driving a tricked-out car. Sure, all of that can be cool, too, but if you're only living your life to please others, it can come off as desperate, even downright annoying, and there's nothing attractive about that.

I learned so much about this from Priscilla. As defined by cultural norms, she's a big girl. And she's absolutely gorgeous. And she's married to an absolutely gorgeous photographer. She's so confident and so well put together that she defines what's hot on her own terms. She gets up every morning and she loves herself, which she shows in the way she does her hair, her makeup, and her always dope outfits. She turns the stereotypes inside out. Because of all that, she is the definition of a bad bitch.

We all gravitate toward people who are super-confident. We want to be in on the secret of what makes them feel so good. What do they know that we don't know? Why is she hav- 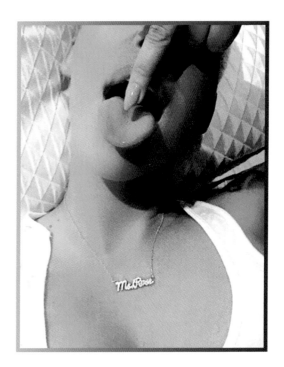 ing such a good time, when we're not? How come she doesn't give a fuck when we do? Because she's a bad bitch, that's why. Sometimes girls worry so much about making the right impression that they forget to have fun. If you're hungry, eat. If there's music and it moves you, dance. A bad bitch is true to herself and doesn't worry or try to make a certain impression. She's too busy living.

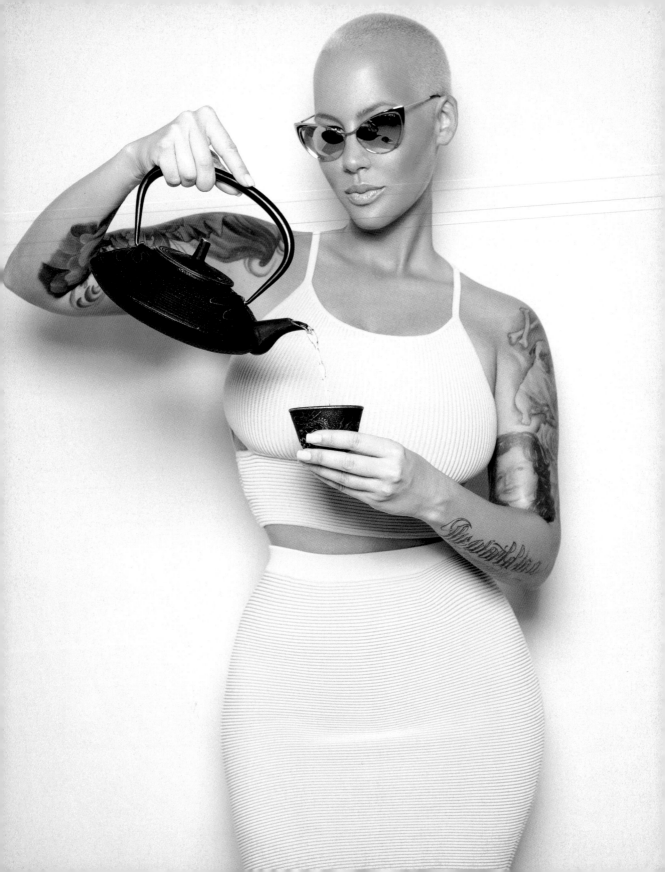

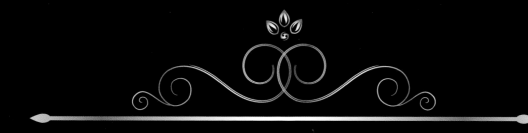

5

Conduct
and
Personality

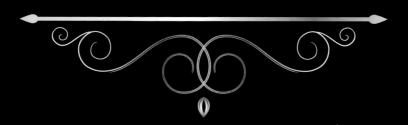

You've perfected your vision. You've put together your hair, makeup, and wardrobe. You've learned to turn life's difficulties into inner strength and channel your self-confidence, no matter what. Now it's time to talk about the impression you create in the world with your conduct and how you carry yourself. It's time to get your behavior in check at Bad Bitch Finishing School. Be warned: good manners are so rare these days that they're often mistaken for flirtation. But that's OK. You know when you're flirting and when you're not. And you don't ever need to lower yourself to other people's standards of behavior; instead, rise to your highest heights, and let others catch up with you. The benefits of making a positive impression are worth the effort. Beauty catches the eye, but personality captures the soul.

Manners simply have to do with being aware of your attitude and behavior and the impression you're making on others. When I'm out anywhere, whether I'm dressed up or dressed down, at a red-carpet event or running to the store, I'm conscious of who's around and how they perceive my actions. This doesn't mean being fake or stuck-up or anything like that. It's about being in control of every situation and the impact you're creating in the world. You'd be amazed at how increasing your attention to detail can make all the difference in your life.

10 Rules to Live By

1 Always hold your head up high when you walk into a room for a full-on, bad-bitch entrance.

2 Always smile. Even when you're not happy on the inside, continue to exude positivity. I wear my heart on my sleeve, so it is very difficult for me to give off an air of happiness when I'm in a totally shitty mood, but I try.

3 Always be extremely nice to those who are serving you in any way. This includes waiters, valets, grocers, beauticians, and the like. There's nothing worse than a rude girl at a restaurant or club. It makes everyone uncomfortable. The staff won't want to serve you properly, and who can blame them? They're just trying to do their jobs, just as you do yours. They don't need your attitude. They're not indebted to you. If you can afford to, always tip well. If you can't afford to tip fairly, don't go out.

4 Always listen more than you speak. That's not to say you should be timid or introverted, but be very aware of your surroundings and everything that's being said, because it ensures you'll always know what's up. I can't stand girls who talk too much or talk over other people. For one thing, it's extremely annoying. For another, they don't give themselves a chance to get to really know anyone else's personality or understand another person's perspective, because they're too busy yapping. Just don't.

5 Always know when to leave a situation or when you're not wanted somewhere. That will make you a real bad bitch. If you see two people talking, walk away. Don't just stand there. Don't linger. Don't hover. Having the confidence to leave at the right moment is much more likely to get you invited back. Sure, I've had those moments, just like everyone else, when I've suddenly felt insecure in a social situation, but I didn't feel the need to stick around. I left, and that made *me* the cool kid.

6 Never hide your needs—including your appetite. Don't avoid getting seconds of food if you're still hungry. From my own experience, a lot of guys find it very attractive. Mind you, this only works if you know how to sit at the table and be respectful of your hosts and servers. Being rude is never OK, no matter how famished you are.

7 Never answer a question too fast. Just relax. Take a deep breath. Pause and allow yourself the time to fully consider what you're going to say. This is very important. What I've learned from a life lived in the spotlight is to always pause and think about something before I say it. When I do interviews, I never give my answer without being sure it's what I really want to put out there. This is a great rule for everyday life, too. You'll be much less likely to say something you'll regret.

8 Don't yell. There's no advantage to raising your voice or trying to battle back and forth with someone, no matter how much cause you have to be upset. You might think you're getting your point across, but you're really not.

9 When you mess up, and we all do, apologize. There's nothing wrong with that. In fact, there's strength in saying you're sorry and moving on. But once you apologize, that's it. You do not repeatedly get down on your hands and knees. If someone is not accepting your sincere apology, then you just keep it moving. It's all you can do.

10 Never be a hater. Complimenting other women can make you look way iller than being bitchy and negative. When you walk into a party and make a big deal out of talking up the hottest girl in the room, you exude pure confidence. I do that all the time. Also, there's no need to be trash-talking. Being from South Philly, I will smack a girl down if she gives me reason to, but I never start a conflict or run my

Being a bad bitch isn't just about being graceful and calculated. It's also about enjoying yourself. Sure, you want to make an impact, but what's the point of being on top of it all if you're so starving and miserable that it's no fun being at the party anyhow? There's nothing sexier than a woman who is living her life to the fullest, but a bad bitch always knows her limit.

You never want to be *that* girl—the drunk girl stumbling out of the club, throwing up, looking a mess. It's not cute. It's not safe. It's very unbecoming for a woman. Hell, it's unbecoming for a guy. It's not a good look on anyone.

If you know you'll be drinking a lot—whether to heal a broken heart or have a wild night—do it in the privacy of your own house with your girlfriends. Be safe, and always drink with people you trust. Don't be afraid to order in food and go off—sometimes it's the most fun you're gonna have. You don't have to worry about your hair or makeup. You can lounge around in your favorite sweats, eating your pizza and chicken wings and drinking too much wine. Go ahead and make

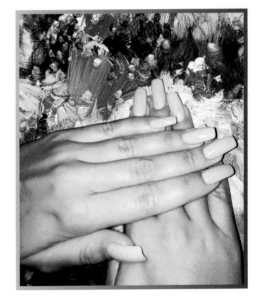

fancy cocktails. You can have a big night without even going outside. Get wasted, if that's fun for you. And if you throw up, it's in your own trash can next to your bed. And when you look like shit the next morning and there's no one there to see you except for your girlfriends, who cares? Sometimes that's the perfect antidote for all that ails you or just a good way to enjoy a day off. Go for it, as long as you're being safe and smart.

Now, when you're out, always keep your composure. Know your limit when it comes to drinks. If you feel a little tipsy, you should stop. You never want to get carried out of the club or do something that you'll regret the next day. And besides, you don't have to get wasted to have a good time. Instead, dance, flirt, laugh.

THE MORNING AFTER

I promise you that I will never try to school you on a subject I have not learned about myself in the University of Hard Knocks. I definitely did my share of drunk-and-disorderly in Philly in my early twenties. Shit, even in recent years. Looking back, it seems ridiculous—getting so blitzed that my friends had to put me in the shower after the club—but that was just a brief period of my life, and I mostly put it behind me long ago. By the time I moved to New York, I was over it. I was in the early stages of living my dream, and I didn't have time to run around like a lunatic. I had to focus.

During my short-lived run as a young wild thing, I pulled my share of embarrassing stunts when drunk. One time, I was leaving a club just as it was letting out, wasted on Crown and Cokes, and I saw a boy I liked. I went to call his name, and as I did so, I walked a little too fast, and I fell and scraped up my elbows and knees. Everyone was outside, and they all laughed at me. The guy looked at me like *Who is this plastered girl?* and didn't even come over to help me up or ask if I was OK. I had my friends pick me up and

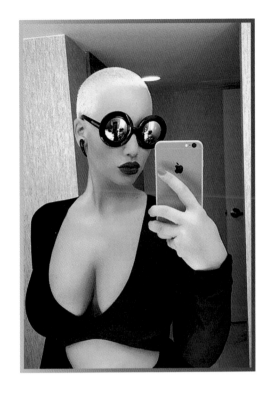

haul me off. I was humiliated. Probably my most embarrassing moment, though, happened one night when I was out at the club with friends on a double date. The lounge cleared a bit, and we were the only two couples on the dance floor. I had just met my date, who was now slow dancing me around. I'd gotten so drunk that my ankle rolled, and I fell right there in front of him on the dance floor. At that time, I thought it was the end of my life. That's when I learned the lesson that getting drunk, and then being stupid, is not a good look.

Normally, I'm a great dancer, and all my friends know it. That only happened because I'd gotten extremely drunk. But to this day, ten years later, when I run into those friends, they always talk about that night. It was so long ago that I can laugh about it with them now. But for the longest time, I was mortified.

The club isn't the only place you need to keep your composure. If you're on a dinner date, especially a first date, absolutely do not drink too much. I think many women do exactly that, because they're nervous, or they're too shy or embarrassed to openly admit they like a guy when they're sober. And then they either look like fools or end up doing things they didn't really want to do because they let the situation get out of control. Don't be *that* girl, either. Neither of those is a good outcome for a date. Of course, if you want to go home with him, go home with him. But if you've kept it to two drinks at most, then you know that's what you actually want to do, instead of having an embarrassing morning after.

OUT THERE FOR THE WHOLE WORLD TO SEE

There was no Instagram back when I was running around South Philly in my early twenties, so it was just my friends and the people at the club who saw my humiliation on my worst nights (including the one time I was so drunk I actually got thrown out of the club). My actions weren't on display for the whole world to see. Sure, we had Myspace back then, but it wasn't anything like the social-media frenzy of today. I've had the luxury of being able to learn from these past experiences without anything incriminating living on the Internet, forever. If you're still acting like a drunken nut in this day and age of instant viral media, it's only a matter of time before something is posted that you really regret. Today women post stuff on social media in a burst of drunken bravado, and that post is never as funny or clever or sexy as they thought it was when they drafted it through the bottom of an empty bottle of booze.

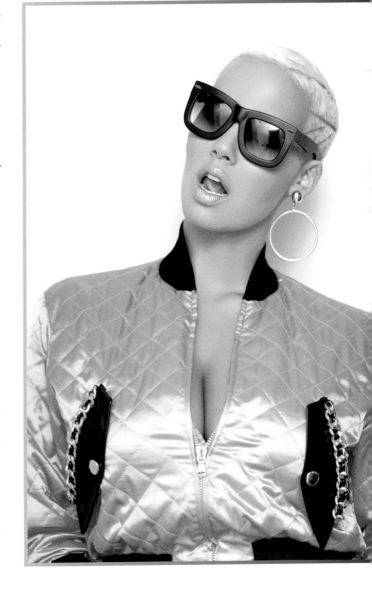

Be even more aware of what you post if you have kids or plan to someday. I'm the proudest MILF out there, and every sexy photo or video I post on the Internet is completely under my control and uploaded by my choice. You may not agree with everything I put out there, but every post comes from my own volition, not from some reckless night.

A Bad Bitch Never Loses Her Cool

Even though I'm older and more on top of things, I've still had moments of bad judgment on social media, which I regretted instantly. There are plenty of things that can cloud your judgment as much as alcohol. Anger. Jealousy. Pain. A bad bitch keeps her real feelings and vulnerabilities to herself, and this is especially true on social media. When you're upset about something, vent to your loved ones—the people you know you can trust—rather than going public with your personal thoughts and feelings. There's a big difference between what's appropriate for your inner circle and the world at large.

If a significant other, a friend, or anyone else has said or done anything—on social media or in everyday life—that is tempting you to go online and rant, stop right there. Take a day or two to sit down and think about what you're going to say or not say. Consider the possibility that your information or understanding of the situation isn't fully correct. Imagine how stupid you'd feel if you later learned that you chewed them out on social media for something that wasn't true.

In this day and age, how you act on social media is an extension of your good—or bad—conduct, so behave responsibly.

This is another moment when it's important to remember that your friends may think they know what's best for you, but that doesn't mean they always have the best advice. That has definitely happened to me. No disrespect to anyone, but sometimes it's easy for other people to be adamant that you need to set the record straight when it really doesn't concern them. The only thing that matters is that your actions are up to your own standards. In private, you can rant and rave as much as you want to, but this is your image, your world, and you control it—nobody else. A bad bitch never loses her cool.

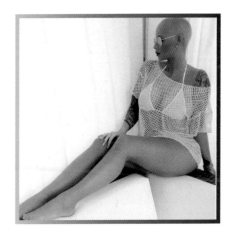

DON'T BE A MEAN GIRL

There's nothing to be gained by making negative comments on anyone's online posts or photos. Don't be a mean girl. You should never leave ignorant and straight-up mean remarks on other girls' pages, critiquing what they're wearing, how their hair is styled, who they're hanging out with, what they're doing in life, or anything like that. Don't even comment on posts that are directly related to you, even if what the person posted is untrue. I know

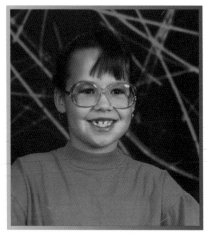
Second grade class picture with glasses and lasers

it's hard to resist. I've seen some people—even celebrities—who respond to every little negative comment about them on the Internet. What a waste of time. First, the people who spread negativity like that are just trolls, desperate for attention. Second, there's no winning against them. There's no setting the record straight. So just let it go. Ignore them, and they'll eventually get bored with harassing you, just like kids finally got bored with teasing me for having glasses when I was a kid.

Another thing is that sometimes, people who treated me badly actually turned out to be nice. You never know what type of day another person is having. So just because someone's mean to you, there's no need to be mean in return. We women are emotional creatures, and we are in danger of constantly getting torn down, not only by men but also by other women. Rise above all of them, and you'll rule both the room and your life.

I know you're going to come back at me with all sorts of times when you didn't start it. Some other girl did. Doesn't matter. If someone posts a nasty comment on your photo or page, just ignore them, and then delete them from your contacts and block them in the future. There's no need to go back and forth and have an argument on social media with someone who obviously just wants to get your attention. They're not worth it.

Trust me, I've been there. I find it's easier never to post comments about other people online, not even nice ones.

A bad bitch is too busy and too fabulous to post comments. Seriously, she is off running her empire, enjoying her life.

She's not checking her phone every two seconds to see what's being said online. Believe me, this philosophy has literally saved my sanity during my divorce. I didn't look. I just didn't. Sure, friends thought they were helping me by telling me what was out there, and it was inevitable that I got exposed to a bunch of nasty stuff. But I never sought it out. I stayed busy, raising my son, writing this book, traveling, making appearances, spending time with my family and friends, building a new life for myself. Muva doesn't have time to suffer.

If you're not posting all the time, your exes and enemies know you aren't giving them a second thought. You're out living it up, having the best day of your life right now. And *that's* the best response of all.

NONJUDGMENT GOES BOTH WAYS

Here's something extremely important. It goes both ways. Do unto others and all that. A bad bitch isn't judgmental of other women. A bad bitch isn't in the business of tearing other women down. Quite the contrary. She appreciates another woman's beauty and differences. A bad bitch always gives credit where credit is due and never fosters unnecessary competition. Before you even think about tearing someone down or calling out another woman, think about your life. Think about things you've done. Reflect on your not-so-shining moments. And put yourself in her shoes. I'll never deny where I came from or the fact that I started out as an exotic dancer. I'm all for a woman making something out of nothing. I'm not going to clown another woman for anything she's done, and I don't appreciate it

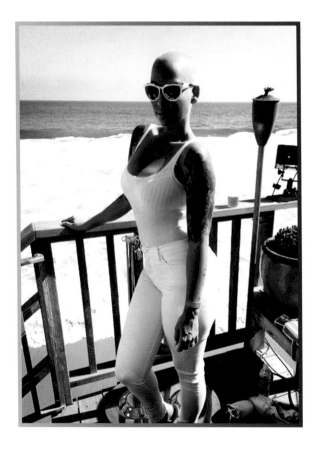

when a woman cops an attitude with me for things that have happened in my past, especially when she's got her own past, too. We're all human.

Life isn't a competition between you and the other women out there. It's really not. There's plenty to go around for everyone—plenty of guys, friends, money, and dreams. It's not like she's diminishing your success just because she's achieved something. Becoming a bad bitch is a process. It doesn't happen overnight. Often, it takes a lot of focus and even more work. If another woman seems to have made more of herself than you have or to have reached a level of success you haven't yet, she's just further along in the process than you are. Don't worry. You'll get there. On the other hand, if another girl is rubbing her success in your face or being competitive with you, a bad bitch

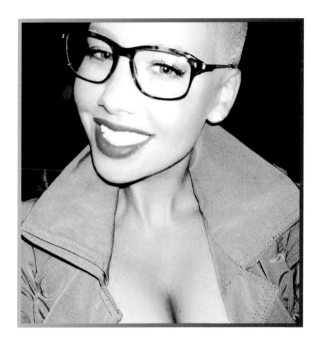

always knows when to keep it moving. So instead of getting jealous or competitive, acknowledge what she's accomplished, and use any negative emotions you might have as fuel to get where you want to go in your own life. It will happen. Maybe it's not your time yet. But it will be soon enough. Have faith, keep working on your goals, and it's inevitable. There's a bad bitch in your future who has everything she wants: you.

Wherever you are in life, having a good attitude and behaving well will give the impression that you're on the top of the world. So use your manners to create an air of success and confidence, even as you're still perfecting your day-to-day reality, and people will be even more likely to help you along your way.

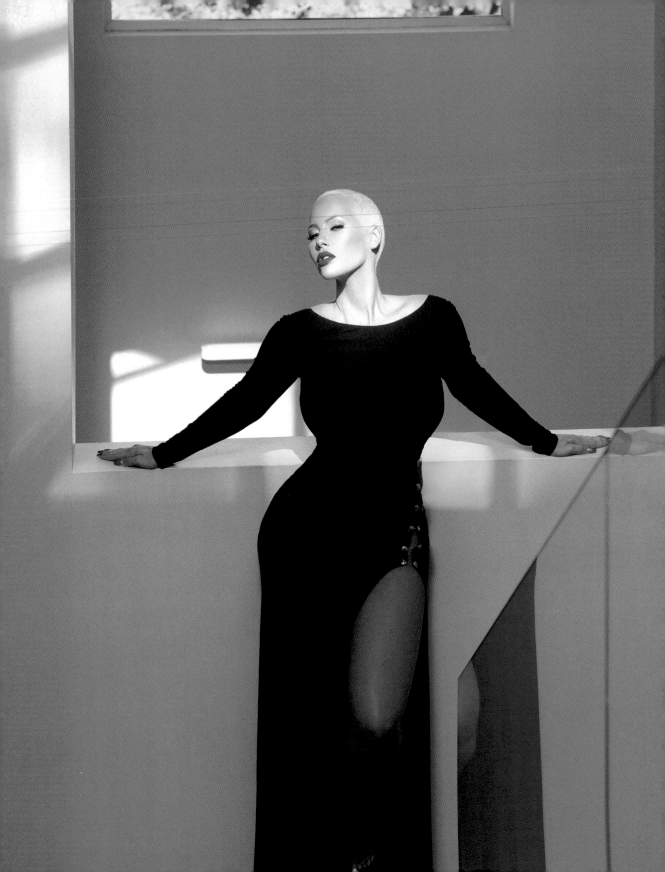

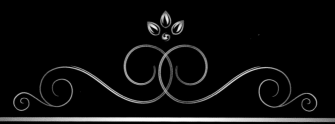

6

FIND
YOUR
PASSION

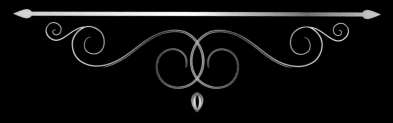

Sometimes you find your passion. Sometimes it finds you. In my case, I got discovered. It took a while, but I never doubted it would happen someday. I always knew I wanted to model and that I would eventually.

When I moved to New York City at age twenty-one, I was also moving closer to my dream of modeling, but I wasn't sure how I was going to break in. I always kept my goals in sight, though. And I did whatever I could to be prepared for the moment when I made it, like staying in shape and having style.

I knew it was in my favor that I was dancing at a really nice club, which attracted very high-end clientele and not just a slew of lonely perverts (not that there aren't plenty of high-end lonely perverts out there, of course). I worked hard, kept my eyes open, and trusted that my moment would come, no matter how long it took.

One night, after I'd been working there for about three years, I noticed a pretty dark-haired woman checking me out while I was onstage. When I was done with my number and out circulating on the floor, she approached me. Up close, I could see she wasn't much older than I was, but she seemed confident and on point.

"You're very beautiful," she said. "Did you ever think about doing music videos?"

I was flattered, but I didn't want to get hustled or lose focus on my real goal. I didn't suspect this could actually lead to a big break. "No, I'm kind of to myself," I said. "I don't know anything about that life. I'm just here, making money, trying to live in New York. It's expensive

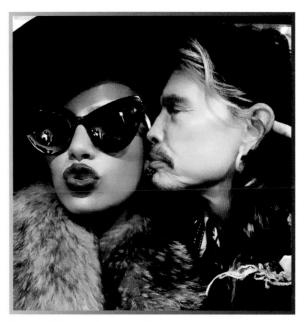

Muva and the legendary Steven Tyler

out here." From what I'd seen so far, most of the girls who danced in videos also had sex with the male singers and rappers, hoping they'd get something out of them or maybe even end up being their girlfriends. I heard these stories all the time. I was not having any of that, and I was determined to find another way to get myself to Hollywood.

But she was persistent. "You could fly out tomorrow, all expenses paid, and you'd get a one-thousand-dollar check," she said.

"What? Are you serious?"

"Very," she said. "My name is Margo Wainwright, and I work for Def Jam. All it will take is one call."

"OK," I said. And that was the beginning.

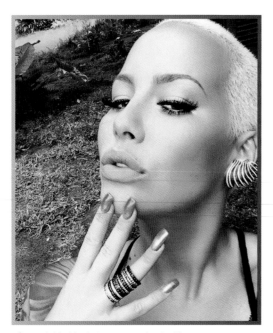

Swaggin' in Maui at my cover shoot with David LaChapelle

She was right. It was just that easy. Not long after that, I flew to Atlanta and did my first video. At the time Margo discovered me, I was wearing a wig, as I normally did when I danced, so I just wore fake hair without mentioning it. The video shoot was for Young Jeezy's "Put On." It was a cool experience, but I was thinking of it as a job, nothing more. I wasn't there to mingle.

I was glad my first video went well, and I was even happier when I got asked back to do the video for Young Jeezy's next single, "Vacation" (that's me in the purple dress and long red hair). Because they'd liked me in a wig for the first video, I opted for that look again the next time around. But I got to thinking after my second video, by wearing a wig, I wasn't really being myself or showing the world my own personal vision of who I really was. I called Margo.

"You know I have a buzz cut underneath this wig I'm wearing, right?"

"No I didn't know that," she said.

"I would really like to rock my buzz cut in the next video," I said. "I feel like it's more me. You found me when I was working, but that's not my everyday look."

"No, I don't think so," she said. "I don't think that's good for a music video."

But I knew my vision was special, and I didn't give up. I was respectful but persistent. I was determined to at least get my chance to show her what I had. "Let me just send you a picture and see if you like it," I said.

When she saw how I looked with a buzz cut, she booked me on the next flight to LA, so I could shoot the video for "What Them Girls Like" by Ludacris with Chris Brown and Sean Garrett. The first shot in that video is looking down on a crowd of dancing girls, with my blond buzz cut at the center of everything.

This was my third video shoot in as many months, and I was starting to get the lay of the land. There was one thing I was very clear on from the beginning. This was a great opportunity for me, and I wasn't going to let anything turn my head.

I knew my vision was special, and I didn't give up. I was respectful but persistent.

It was a cool experience, but I was very professional. There were a lot of rappers running around, but I wasn't about to go there. I was careful to radiate this attitude: *I am here to do a job. I am a beautiful model, and you're going to treat me as such. Don't talk to me inappropriately.* And they did respect that, every single one of them.

I've seen too many girls who have a very different agenda when they're around rappers or any kind of famous men. They go in there thinking,

Maybe if I have sex with this guy, he'll do something for me. It's stupid as fuck. And those girls ruin it for girls like me. I just wanted to look beautiful and be on TV. There's nothing wrong with that, by the way. It's certainly a fun way to make good money. It's just important, in situations like that, or in any situation, really, to be strategic and think about the long run. There's a time and a place for everything. I'm all for girls feeling free to sleep with whoever they want to, but a moment like that isn't about getting some. It's about being a bad bitch and laying the groundwork for more connections and income.

After I did that video, everything started happening for me. And it was my look that did it, too. That's when everyone noticed me and

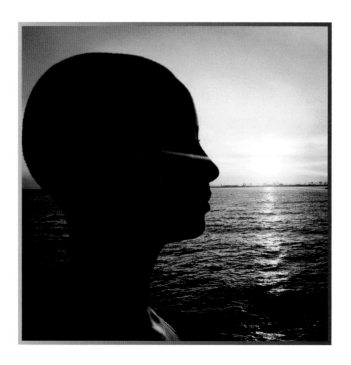

started asking around, "Who's the bald girl in the Ludacris and Chris Brown video?"

I could feel a kind of a buzz building immediately. Having Margo on my side definitely helped, too. Not long after that, I met Def Jam cofounder Russell Simmons. And that was my *big* break. While I was right there in his office, he picked up his phone, called Katie Ford, and got me a meeting—just like that. When I walked into Ford Models, they signed me that same day. So, yes, thank you, Russell.

A Bad Bitch Asks for Help

Soon I was getting plenty of modeling work. I was twenty-five, and I decided it was time to take a leap of faith and make my move to live my Hollywood dream. There was just one problem. I had about fifteen hundred dollars in my bank account, and when I found my perfect Hollywood apartment, my rent was three thousand dollars a month. I knew this was where I was meant to live, and I wasn't about to let a little thing like money stop me.

I went to the owner of the building, and I broke it down for him. "Look, I want to live here," I said. "I really don't have the money right now, but I have a few things lined up. If you give me a chance, for two months, I promise I'll pay all the money I owe you, plus a couple of months in advance."

After I made my case, I knew enough to shut up and let him decide what he wanted to do. I stood there, feeling a little nervous, until he gave me a big smile. "OK," he said.

"Really?" I said. "I'll make it up to you, I promise."

"In the Jewish religion, we have a tradition where you do something for someone and expect nothing in return," he said.

I'll never forget that leap of faith he took on me. He let me move into his building in Hollywood, and just like I'd promised him, within two months, I was able to pay him back all the money I owed him and pay the full rent every month. Not only that, but maybe six months later, my career had really taken off, and I had a shitload of money. My landlord ended up asking me if he could borrow ten thousand dollars from me. Of course, I lent him the money. He'd done me a solid, and I was happy to help him. He was really serious about paying me back. He copied his ID for me, and he gave me a note stating his intentions, which he signed.

And you know what? I never got that money back. I never even saw him again after that. I don't know exactly what happened to him, but he left that building, and eventually, I moved away, too. That was OK with me, though. I didn't even want the money from him. It was more like he had done something for me, and then I had done something for him, so it all worked out. It wasn't about the money anymore. He really trusted me, and that meant a lot to me. It kind of set the tone for my new life in Los

Angeles, like it gave me confidence because I could tell everything was going to work out the way I wanted it to.

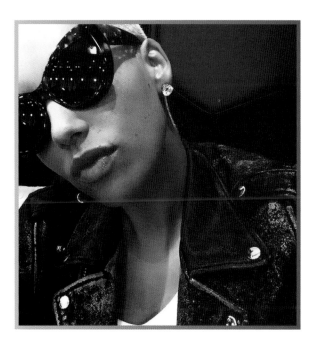

So don't hesitate to ask for something. It's impossible to follow your passion without enlisting help from others along the way, and daring to ask for assistance when you need it is actually a form of strength. I still employ this philosophy today. How do you think I got the incredibly fabulous David LaChapelle to shoot the cover of my book? That's right, I asked him. He was happy to do it, which I still can't get over. Life is amazing. We just have to do everything in our power to help make it so.

THE ONE RULE THAT REALLY MATTERS

There's only one rule that *really* matters when you're honing in on your passion: be authentic. Don't act like someone you're not, or pretend you're interested in accomplishing something you don't really care about, just because you think it's what you should be doing, or what will make other people like you.

I may have consciously chosen how to do my makeup and what to wear, but every single detail of my look and life is a direct expression of who I really am. If you watch the first music videos I appeared in, you can see my long red wig. Long hair is pretty, don't get me wrong, but

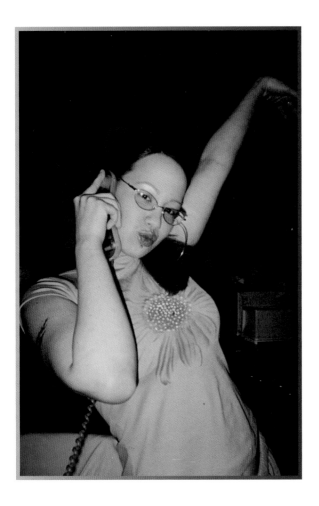

I felt I looked like every other girl in every other rap video, soap opera, or car commercial. That's not really me. I didn't get discovered until I was confident rocking a look that's true to who I am inside—fierce, edgy, and beautiful.

I may have moved up in the world, but I'm still the same girl from South Philly. That's why my look and persona don't feel artificial. Because they're

The age changed, but the pose stayed the same. Here I am at one of my girlfriend's houses when I was sixteen.

not. I have always been true to myself and stayed true to my values. This is so important. People know when you're faking it. They know when a woman isn't being herself, and it comes off as desperate. That's not to say you can't aspire to become something more than where you started out in life. In fact, that's exactly what you should do, but working toward your true, ideal self is

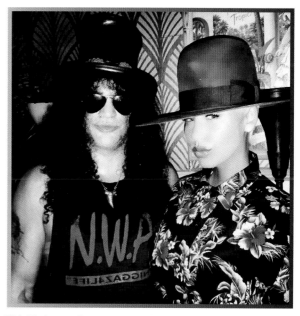

With Slash, one of my heros, from Guns n' Roses—my favorite band of all time!

much different than masquerading as something you're not. You know yourself. Be *that* self. Don't try to be anyone else.

The entire world won't approve of the self you are. But you know what? Fuck them. You'll find your people, and you'll know they're the ones who really like you for you. If you're acting like someone you're not and people get a whiff of that, they're gonna want to steer clear of you anyhow. They're certainly not going to help you make your goals happen. If you're comfortable with yourself, you'll give off positive energy, and people will want to be around you and get in line with where you're going in your life. Learn to love yourself and everything about you, and people will see how lovable you are, too. While life isn't a popularity contest, using your true self to

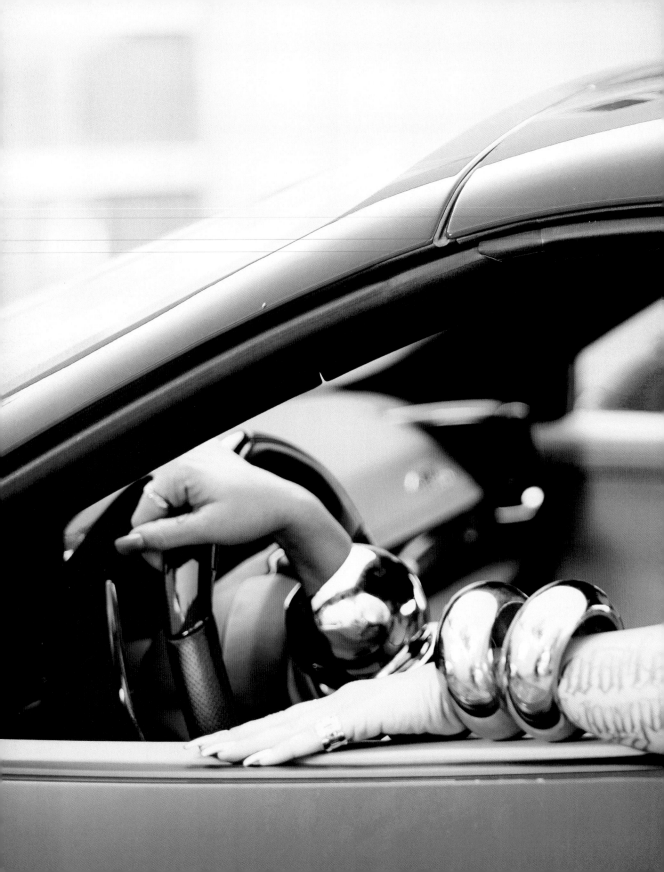

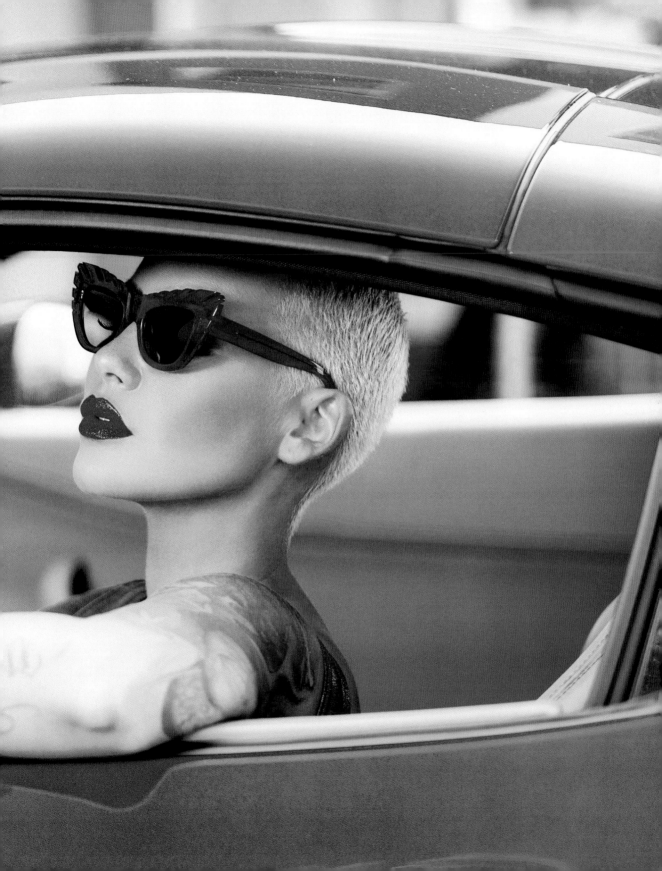

enlist the support of others will go far toward getting that job you know would be perfect for you, or that loan you need to start your dream business, or doing anything else you just have to do.

INVENT YOURSELF FROM THE INSIDE OUT

I'm aware that not everyone is born knowing what she wants to do in life, like I was. That's OK. It gives you the chance to invent yourself from

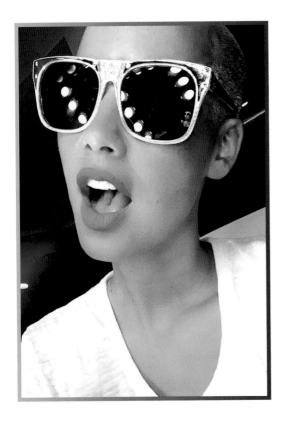

the inside out. And it doesn't have to be a process where you go off to the top of a mountain and meditate for a year to uncover the answer, either. If you stay open, you can find inspiration anywhere and everywhere. Maybe you're watching TV, and you see a program about a real estate agent, or a personal trainer, or a chef, and you get this feeling like that's what you're really meant to be doing. Once you uncover your dream, learn more about what the job really entails and how much schooling or training is involved to get there. Then, create a plan for making it happen.

If inspiration doesn't come to you that easily, try browsing the self-help section of your local bookstore to see all of the resources out there that could guide you. Or even just think about the people in your life who seem really happy and satisfied. What works for them and why? Maybe it's not a new job that will bring you joy, but a new hobby or a new artistic endeavor. No matter what you decide to pursue, just remember you don't have to explain it or justify it to anyone. Your passion is your true calling in life, whether others like it or not.

No matter what you decide to pursue, just remember you don't have to explain it or justify it to anyone. Your passion is your true calling in life, whether others like it or not.

DEMAND THE ATTENTION

So much of making your dream life happen is about getting seen, whether it's by the person interviewing you for a job, the clients you need to impress during a meeting, or the customers you want to attract to your venture. According to my mom, I've always had the ability to make people take notice, even when I was way too young to know anything about self-confidence or composure. "Amb, I don't know what it is, but when you walk into a room, you demand attention." I've heard her say that since I was small.

I don't go in and announce myself. I don't say, "Hey, everyone, I'm here." It's just a natural poise I have, almost more of an inner strength and stillness, and I honestly feel like that's why I've been able to get what I want. It helped me when I was dancing, and I definitely learned how to cultivate it more over the years. It helped me to get discovered and break into music videos. And it helped me translate my music video work into a modeling career and everything else.

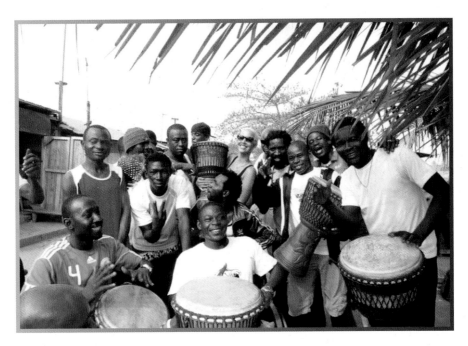

Visiting Ghana in 2011—I am truly passionate about helping people, and this was one of the most inspiring trips I have ever taken.

Set a Goal and Make It Happen

I've found that the best approach is to have one specific goal in mind that's challenging but attainable. If you want something too general, it can be hard to see the steps you must take to get there. You might say your goal is to be rich. Sure, we'd all like to be rich. But what does that even mean? What does that look like? How do you get there, if you're barely making ends meet now? Instead, set your sights on something specific and attainable: getting your own apartment, buying a new car, or paying down all of your credit-card debt. Then you'll know exactly how much money you need to achieve your goal, and you can work toward making that happen.

Once you've set your goal, don't let anything get in your way. People will say no. That's part of life. People may even say you're not good enough, or pretty enough, or skinny enough, or smart enough. I've certainly heard all of those things before. It doesn't make them true. Look at Oprah Winfrey. She came from nothing. She doesn't look like a model. But nobody kept her down. She kept pushing and achieving and striving to be better, and now, she's gorgeous and powerful and on top of the world. She owns a whole channel. Oprah's a bad bitch.

I have an inner bad bitch, and it runs the show. You have one, too. You just have to strengthen her, and the world will be at your fingertips. What we're trying to capture in this book are the tools every woman needs to find whatever *that thing* is inside herself that allows her to live the best life possible. Learn to trust yourself and pursue your goals relentlessly, and you can't help but unleash your inner bad bitch on the world. It's inevitable.

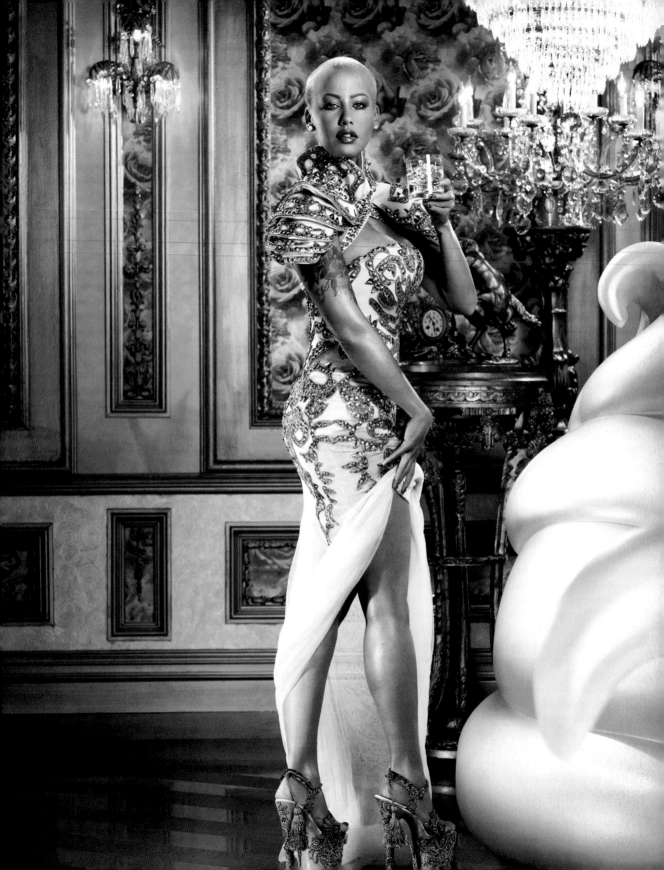

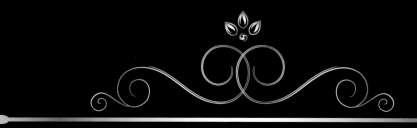

7

MONEY
AND
YOUR CAREER

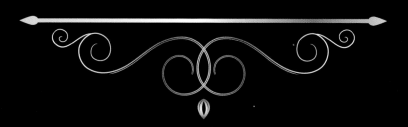

Any woman who has her finances together is an automatic bad bitch, for sure. It's all well and good to learn this stuff and take it down to the club, but I want bigger and better for you. What I really want is to get you to a place where you have the confidence to win at whatever corner of the world you choose to dominate. Whether you're a stay-at-home mom, a hairstylist, or the CEO of a Fortune 500 company, you should be on top of your game. And too many women aren't. It's almost like they're afraid of their own potential, or maybe no one ever showed them what they're capable of achieving, or they continuously let a man keep them down. Well, it's time to change that once and for all. You don't have to ask anyone's permission to take control of your finances and make your wallet work for you.

Being an exotic dancer was basically my own version of business school. When you are in a line of work where you are literally persuading men to take their hard-earned cash out of their pockets and put it into your hands, you'd better learn some things about money, the art of acquiring it, and the importance of managing it well. I learned all of this while I was making my way out in the world, bad-bitch style. I had to work for everything I have, and I didn't have anyone to handle my money or my career, so I had to be smart. And now, I'm going to pass my wisdom along to you, so you can up your game in your professional life, or even just in the realm of your own personal finances.

POWER, PLAIN AND SIMPLE

I'm not going to lie—I think much of my inner bad bitch came from being an exotic dancer. I learned how to seduce a man at a very young age and in a way that many women in their thirties and forties don't even know how to do, and I turned it into a good living. I'm not ashamed of that at all, because it's power, plain and simple, and it's been an incredibly valuable tool in my life, which I continue to draw on in business and love.

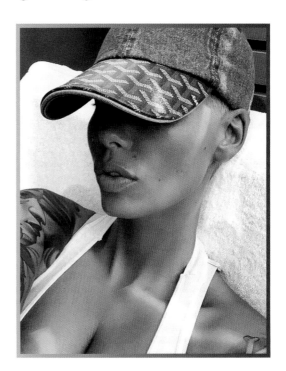

When you're hungry or you need the cash from tips *that day* to pay your rent in the morning, you get good at seduction. You don't have the time to be self-conscious or feel undeserving. You have to learn, quickly, to sell yourself as simply the best. Dancing isn't about selling a view of your body. It's

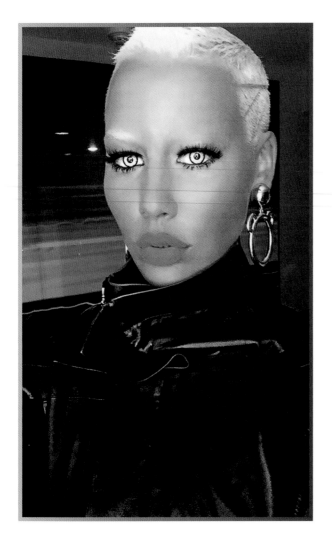

about selling your confidence. It took me years to learn how to master the art of seduction, but once I got it down, I could use it anywhere: at the club where I worked, sure, but also in front of the camera as a model and even today in business meetings.

I know you're probably thinking you don't have years to practice and learn all of this. You have a job interview tomorrow. Your car payment is due this week. You want to be a bad bitch now. Well, let me teach you a few basics that can go a long way toward making the impression you want to make.

And then you can practice and refine your technique going forward, just like I did. I'm still learning and perfecting, and I plan to keep doing so for the rest of my life. Now it's your turn.

The first tool is eye contact. But it's more than that, too. When you're in a job interview or a meeting, look at the people on the other side of the table like you're in love with them. Obviously, this doesn't mean you should flirt with them or do anything sexual or suggestive. I'm simply talking about bringing the same kind of focus and intensity to your interactions as you would if you were talking to someone you loved deeply. Stare into their eyes, really listen to everything they say, and let them speak more than you do. This can take you far, especially when it comes to business and relationships. Ask them questions, and draw them out on topics that interest them, so you'll know what they enjoy and care about. That way, when it comes time to make them feel like they want to be in a relationship with you—whether it's a business transaction or a date—you'll nail it, because you'll have the knowledge to make them feel really special.

Pull them in, and get to know them. If you just sit there and talk about yourself the whole time, you're missing a real opportunity. As women, we often like to talk about ourselves and our feelings, but it's always good to learn about the people we meet, too. Other people like attention, and like to feel appreciated, just like we do. Sometimes making it seem like you're giving other people what they want is a great way to make them want to give you what you want.

I know I was lucky to work at really nice clubs in Philly and New York, where every girl was sweet and beautiful. I made a bunch of friends, the guys behaved themselves, and the security was on point. I had so much fun, and I made so much money. Part of me misses it every day. In some ways, it was the best time of my life. Even though it was my job, I got to make my own schedule, and I actually looked forward to going into the club. It honestly felt more like a social gathering than a night at work.

At the start of my shift, as soon as I went into the dressing room and began getting ready, I always had the most fun. The other girls and I were like sisters, and whenever we saw each other, we gave big hugs and checked in. While doing each other's makeup, we laughed and joked and listened to sexy, upbeat music that put us in the mood.

We looked out for each other, too. One of the girls would go out and survey the scene, then report back. "A bachelor party just walked in," she'd call out. "Let's go make some money!"

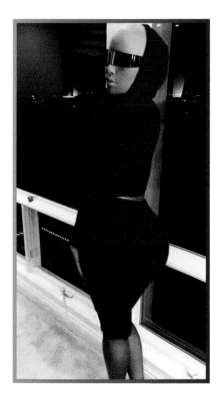

We'd all whoop and shout and quickly put on our finishing touches in the long mirror before we went out into the club together as one big unit. We never tried to undermine the other girls or take all of the business for ourselves. There was enough money to go around, and we were happy to support each other and to share. It really was a sisterhood. This is a good lesson, no matter what line of work you're in. Make friends with your coworkers instead of being competitive, and you'll not only enjoy the job more, but you'll be more successful, too. Being nice pays, literally.

I learned another important lesson while I was dancing. It's good to find a mentor and get her to teach you the ropes. I'd first tried dancing when I was fifteen, but I didn't like it. I was way too young—illegal, in fact. I wasn't in the right mind-set. It was too much for me. When I tried it again at eighteen, on my first night, I met Autumn. That right there made all the difference. She was a gorgeous petite redhead who was about thirty years old, and she taught me everything I needed to know to be safe and make money. She taught me how to give a lap dance appropriately. She taught me that a lot of men were going to try to take me home but that I should never go. She taught me that I was beautiful and that if I knew how to talk to men, it would be enough to allow me to earn a ton of money. I would make bank, and then I would go home and pay my bills, and that would be it. Under her guidance, I came

Make friends with your coworkers, instead of being competitive, and you'll not only enjoy the job more, but you'll be more successful, too.

to know my worth, and I came to know what I would and wouldn't do. And once I was clear on both of these facts, I never let anyone cross the line with me. My whole experience as an exotic dancer was positive and profitable, largely because of Autumn. I've taken this lesson forward and found mentors in other areas of life, and I would strongly encourage you to do the same.

Autumn and my whole experience dancing taught me how to be personable. It taught me how to flirt. It taught me how to laugh it off when someone said something rude to me, instead of getting offended or losing control of the situation. It taught me how to get what I want when I want it. It taught me to make the most of any opportunity. And the truth is, this kind of unwavering self-confidence is just as useful for a bad bitch in business as it is in a relationship. Because, let me tell you, men are the same. In the bedroom. In the boardroom. I can go to a CEO of a billion-dollar company and get what I want. And I'm not being fake. I'm just revealing myself to him in order to let him like me. I'm drawing him in by opening up everything and getting to know him and what he wants out of the situation. It feels good for the other person, too. And it's not a lie, I actually do like getting to know other people and giving them what they want, as long as it's not anything I don't want to give them. I just always make sure to get what I want, first and foremost. This is the real potential of learning to be a bad bitch.

SELF-PROTECTION IS POWER

Here's the thing: sometimes you have to win people over. When I was dancing, there were guys who didn't want to like me. In fact, they were really mean to me. Being up onstage was only a small part of the night.

When we started our shift, we'd go onstage for the men to see our beauty before we went to talk to them. And then, after a song or two, we'd get down and make a round of the club, basically hanging out with guys and trying to get them to spend money on us. We always made some tips when we were onstage, but the real money was from lap dances. We wanted to make the most money in the least amount of time, so we got really good at reading which guys in the club had money and were willing to part with it. This meant looking for the guys who were spending a lot of money on drinks, the ones who weren't just nursing a bottle of beer and tipping girls one dollar per number.

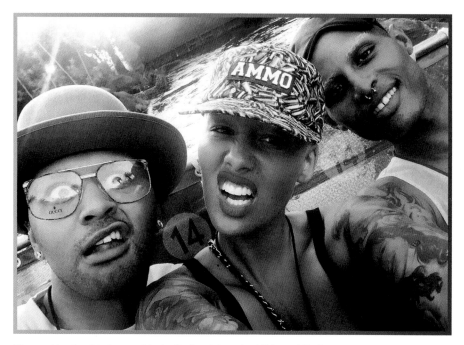

Muva and her two fabulous assistants, Benji and Joseph, at Universal Studios.

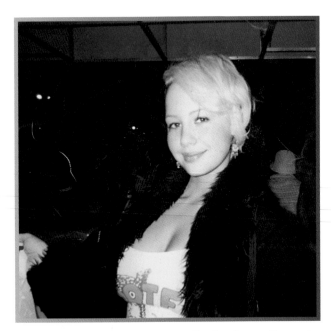

I worked at Hooters when I was eighteen. Here I am in my uniform and natural hair (well, not my natural color, but no weaves).

But even as good as I got at reading people, sometimes I didn't get the response I wanted. I remember stopping near a guy who'd obviously been checking me out from across the room. I gave him a flirty smile.

He practically growled at me. "You're not my type," he said. "Get away from me."

I really needed money, so I didn't have the luxury of getting bent out of shape. And so I turned it around. "You really hurt my feelings," I said. "I came over here because you're really cute, and I thought you were a nice guy. I just thought that maybe we could talk or something like that."

I could see the shift on his face immediately. "Oh, OK. I'm actually sorry for saying that," he said. "I really didn't mean it. I was just being a dick."

Just like that, I made even the dudes with the toughest exteriors soften up. Even when I couldn't read them at first, I always made sure to understand their wants. Eventually, I became one of the most popular dancers at the club, because I'd appeal to them by being myself, inside and out. I

A Bad Bitch Makes Sure
All Her Bills Are Paid

A bad bitch makes sure all her bills are paid before she spends money on anything else. And she spends her money wisely. For years, I had to make my money stretch as far as I could, so I bought almost all my clothes at thrift stores. You can find some really cool gems that barely cost anything. For jewelry, go to the beauty-supply store and buy the cutest costume pieces you can find. For *cheap*. If you are going to drop some serious money on anything, invest in shoes or accessories, because they last, and in keeping your hair done, because it's such an important part of the first impression you make. And if you can't, then find a workaround, like I did. I've been doing my own hair for the past thirteen years. Just think of the thousands of dollars I've saved.

A Bad Bitch Has Her Priorities Straight

I know talking about your finances may sound like a drag, but it's not. It's a crucial step in making your dreams come true. Be patient. It can take time to get your finances in order, but it's always worth it. That's why a strong set of priorities is so important. Whenever you're tempted to buy the extra handbag or drink, ask yourself if losing that money is going to help you be the person you want to be or live the life you want to lead.

If you're going to make a move or start a business or buy a car, you can't always be going out. You have to save. Even if your friends want to go out—and they will, believe me—you can't just decide you're going to go along with them. You've got to remember that you've got a plan and you're sticking to it. This doesn't mean you can't have any fun. Just be up-front with your friends about your goals and priorities. If they're your real friends, they'll understand and want to support you in any way possible.

This is another area where being nice can go a long way. Back in Philly and New York, when I was saving what little money I had, I was super-friendly to all the club owners and door guys every time I went out. Before long, I knew everyone, and they let me into the clubs for free. This was a lifesaver. Paying a ten- or twenty-dollar cover was expensive. Even when I saved the cost of admission, buying drinks added up, too.

I learned how to have fun for cheap. A couple of bottles of wine and your favorite dance music can be an instant party. Have your girlfriends over for a spa night. If your mom's an incredible cook like mine is, have her make your childhood favorite and invite your ladies over for a feast. Good times can be had for almost no money.

It helps if you have friends who are also goal-oriented, because they'll totally get it. We'll get into my thoughts on choosing your friends a little later, but for now, I'll just say that if your friends are also bad bitches, they will support you and help you achieve everything you want in life. Not only that, but they'll also be focused on what they've got going on in their own lives. So they won't always be distracting you by wanting to do stuff that's going to slow you down.

Even if you're perfectly happy with where you are right now, having your finances in order will make everything else easier and less stressful. And it will allow you to afford those little extras that will be a real treat for you—whether it's that pair of boots you've got your eye on or a vacation. It's your dream, so dare to dream it, and don't stop until you've made it a reality.

Unfortunately, I see strong, balanced finances as a challenge for many women. I don't believe in making generalizations (like "women are impulsive"), but I definitely have seen girlfriends spend money on stuff they can't really afford or don't really need. Maybe it's because we are emotional creatures, and we like to make ourselves and the people

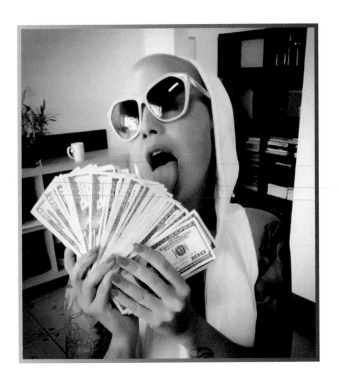

we care about happy. That's more than OK if everything's taken care of and your bills are paid. You can do whatever the hell you want. If your electricity is turned off because you just had to get your hair done, then that is a problem.

I'm actually glad I had those ten years of learning how to manage my money when there wasn't much to manage, because it gave me the tools to run my own business now. Every day is a different adventure, and there's always something happening to keep me on my toes—but I know how to keep myself in check.

LISTEN MORE THAN YOU TALK

Co-parenting my son with my ex while also juggling all my different business ventures means I've got to be efficient and speedy. I don't have the time to agonize over any of my decisions. I have to know what's best for me and my family, and I have to know it right away. This is why I'm so glad I had all those years of learning how to handle myself before I got to where I am today.

Now, when my people come to me with a decision that needs to be made, I'm careful to listen more than I talk, so I can learn everything I need to know about all sides of the situation. And then I look inside for the answer. I always know right away, in my gut, the best step for me.

Sometimes they can't believe I've made up my mind so quickly, and they try to get me to take more meetings or to deliberate a little while longer. But I'm always clear on the fact that when I know, I know. The same goes for situations in which something isn't quite working out in business or in life. If the right solution hasn't been found yet, I don't rush into anything. But when I'm not happy with something, I

> *When my people come to me with a decision that needs to be made, I'm careful to listen more than I talk, so I can learn everything I need to know about all sides of the situation.*

have the confidence to speak up right away and get it fixed. And I want this confidence for you, too. The good news is that it's something you can learn how to do.

I truly believe we all know much more than we give ourselves credit for. Just think of all the times you suspected a friend, lover, or boss was being shady, but you didn't act on your suspicions because you wanted to be nice and give them the benefit of the doubt, or you were afraid you'd look foolish if you were wrong, only to have them go ahead and betray or disrespect you in some equally upsetting way. And how much worse did it feel because you'd known all along not to trust them? And yet you'd doubted yourself and, in a way, given them more credit than you gave yourself.

Always listen to that first suspicion, and act on it. Let me tell you, when I haven't done so in the past, I've been hurt badly. And a bad bitch doesn't let herself get hurt in the same way twice. I always trust my instincts now. If you can start doing so, too, you'll have far greater happiness and security.

The best thing you can do is start listening to yourself more than you listen to anyone else in your life. I know it can be tempting to go to your family and friends when you're dealing with a big decision or a stressful situation and ask them for their advice. It almost seems less scary to make a stand if you're doing whatever everyone else is telling you to do. But I think that's a really dangerous position to be in.

Yes, the people in your life have your best interests at heart, but they're not you. They don't know what's *really* important to you or what it's like to *be* you. They don't have that same vision of the true you inside them, like you have it inside yourself.

Now, I'm not only responsible for myself. I have a whole team of people working for me, and that's another level of responsibility with its own challenges and rewards. To be a boss, you have to inspire a certain level of trust in your employees, but you also have to harness the power of respectful influence. They have to want to work hard for you. If you display your force in a positive way, it actually encourages people to put in the effort for you. They know you can take care of them by keeping the whole empire running, and they know you'll be in charge of any problem that may arise. Sometimes this means dealing with some uncomfortable situations, but you're the boss, and you can handle it. Remember, friendship is friendship, and business is business. If your employees are not doing their jobs, you have to pull them aside for a talk. Don't yell. Be respectful, but also be firm. Let them know what they're doing wrong, and bring them into the process of finding a solution. If they make the same mistake again, consider giving them a time out.

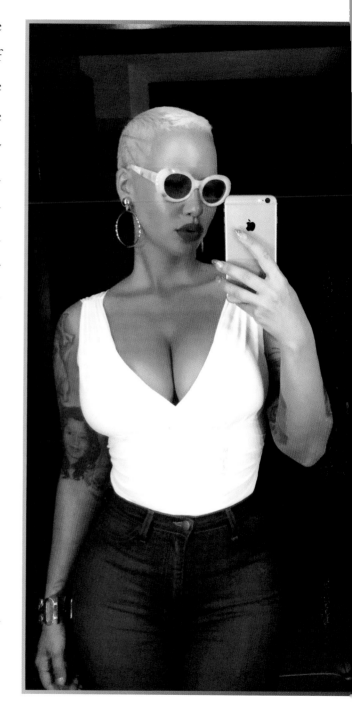

Send them home, and ask them to think about what they want and if this job is it.

Sometimes being a boss means being a referee. Again, it's really important to be respectful and fair but also to be firm. I had two employees who just could not get along. I started watching their interactions, and I saw that one employee was bullying the other. When it was clear that this was really what was happening, I sat the bully down and had a talk about what I'd seen. I wouldn't stand for any denial or excuses. I made my commandment: "Get it together, or I'm sending you home." She got the message loud and clear, and now everyone gets along great.

LEARN FROM YOUR MISTAKES

When I met my bestie, Priscilla Ono, it was bad-bitch love at first sight. Ever since then, we've been inseparable, so we decided we should start a business. *We're together every day. We love and trust each other. So, let's make money together, too.*

We immediately knew what kind of business it was going to be. Having both grown up broke and style-obsessed in low-income neighborhoods with limited fashion resources, we wanted to bring hot clothes to poor girls of all sizes. So we started our online clothing boutique, Rose and Ono.

From the beginning, it was an equal partnership, and the business grew organically. We each put in an equal amount of seed money. We both did everything ourselves and worked equally hard to figure out what we needed to do to make our business a success and then get it done.

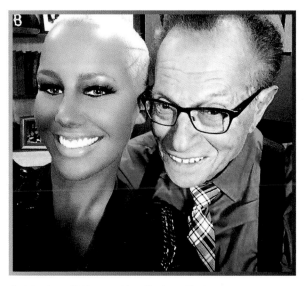

An interview with the man himself—Larry King!

I thought back to the lessons I'd learned earlier in my career and decided to get some expert advice right at the beginning. I searched for online retailers with a vibe we liked and contacted a bunch of them persistently, until a few people got back to me. You'd be surprised how far good manners and a positive attitude can go. Even though I didn't have anything to offer them in return, several of these business owners were happy to get on the phone and give me advice about the do's and don'ts of this kind of enterprise. That saved us so much time and money, and I'm incredibly grateful to them for their generosity and helpfulness.

Once we had a list of what we needed to get started, Priscilla and I went to the courthouse to get our business licenses. We used the money we'd put in to hire a website designer, acquire our first batch of clothes—which we picked out ourselves—and get the site up and running. Throughout this process, we stayed crystal-clear on our mission statement; it was defi-

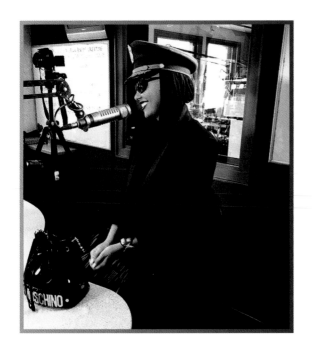

nitely important for Rose and Ono to be a representation of us and our personal style. It was also very important that we carried plus-size clothes. Right after I had my son, none of my clothes fit me anymore. I'd never been plus-size, and I didn't know how to dress. I looked to Priscilla for guidance, and she helped me out. That experience was a real eye-opener for me. Both of us wanted to make sure no girl was left out.

While we both had the same vision and loved and respected each other very much, it wasn't always easy. I'm very strong-minded, and Priscilla is very sensitive. Just because we were best friends, that didn't mean we didn't argue like crazy at times. We both had money invested, and we both thought we knew the best way to succeed. A typical fight was for me to adamantly state my opinion until Priscilla started to cry and ran out of the room. "Amber, this is fucking bullshit," she'd yell at me on her way out. And I'd be thinking, *Suck it up. We've got a business to run.*

We both got mad at times, but we never, ever gave up on the website or each other. We never went through a period where we didn't talk every day. It takes a lot for me to get emotional. I'm very practical. But I'll admit that sometimes my strong opinions cloud my clarity, so it was good to have Priscilla's more intuitive and emotional point of view in the mix, too. We balanced each other out. And once our tempers had cooled down, we never allowed ourselves to take any of this personally. This was business. Our friendship would never be threatened by anything that happened at work.

I'll admit it. I was wrong sometimes. After the orders started rolling in, I felt it was ridiculous for Priscilla and me to be the ones mailing out clothes when we were so busy with our own careers. So I pushed for us to get a fulfillment company to ship orders for us. We ended up spending more money on that than we were making on the orders that came in. Looking back, we probably should have done more research on the fulfillment company we used. It was definitely a learning process.

In the end, we realized we weren't making enough money to justify the time and energy we were taking away from our own careers. At the same time, I could post a picture of myself in a pair

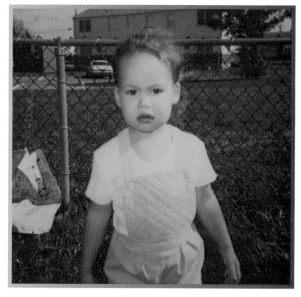

Tell me I don't look like Bash. This was taken when I was two years old, playing in the park in Fort Dix, New Jersey, where my dad was stationed at the time.

> *There's nothing better than having an idea, bringing it to fruition, and having other people tell you how much their lives have been improved by what you've created.*

of our sunglasses, and they'd sell out that day. So we began to focus on just sunglasses. Then I decided to start my own sunglasses line. At first, I was a little worried that Priscilla would think I was giving up on our vision. But she totally understood, and she would never hold me back from having my own venture, just like I would never hold her back from having her own makeup line. Like I've said, business is business. And when we realized our partnership was interfering with our friendship, which we didn't want at all, we finally decided to pursue our own careers instead of a shared business and remain best friends.

Starting your own business is definitely a lot of work, but it's so rewarding. There's nothing better than having an idea, bringing it to fruition, and having other people tell you how much their lives have been improved by what you've created. This sense of personal satisfaction keeps me going on the late nights when I'm exhausted from juggling so much all day and still have to stay up going over business decisions.

My number one job at the moment is being a mom to my son, and that means that when I get home from meetings or auditions, I devote all my time and energy to teaching him, playing with him, and giving him all my attention. Then it's time for dinner, a bath, a bedtime story, and a good-night snuggle. By the time I've wrapped up my favorite part of my

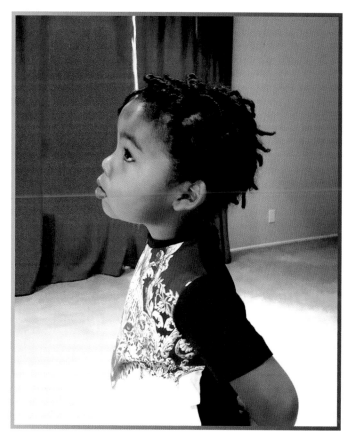

The love of my life, Sebastian.

day, I'm often answering my e-mails and texts around nine o'clock at night or later. Not to mention the nighttime appearances that are a part of my life, while my mom stays home with my son. It's more than a full-time job, but I love it all so much. I wouldn't have it any other way. Live your best life, and you'll go to bed exhausted and rewarded at the end of every day, ready to get up and do it all again tomorrow.

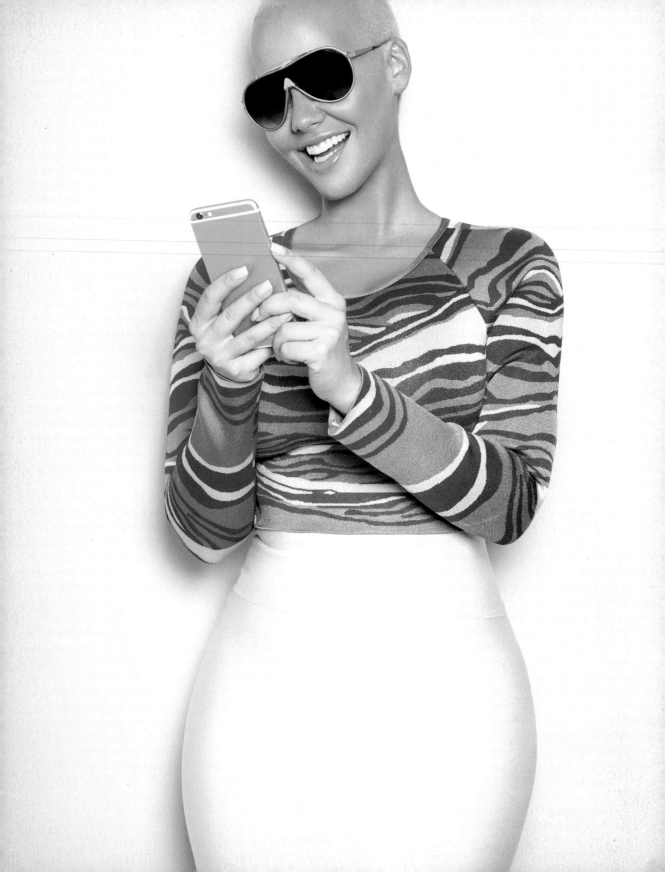

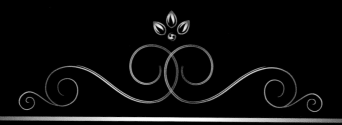

8

FRIENDS

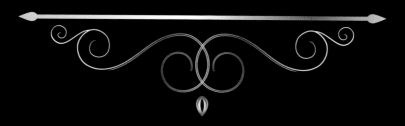

Now it's time to evaluate your crew. You've got it going on, and you're busy building your empire. The last thing you need is a girlfriend who's falling-down drunk or being mean and nasty to everyone. One way to help make sure you're always being the best bad bitch you can be is to recognize and draw on the strengths of your friends. Some friends are down when you need to drink too much wine and laugh your ass off, and others are the perfect strong partners to start a business with, and yet others are great at being your wingwoman when you've got your eye on a fine man.

Not only will this chapter cover the basics of how to assemble a kickass circle of friends, but it will also talk about how to clean house when someone is bringing you down and how to be a good friend to the real sisters in your life. If you're hanging on to a friend from back in the day who clearly has a different vision of life from yours, here's some tough love: just because you've known someone for what seems like forever, that doesn't necessarily mean she still fits into your life. People grow apart, and that's OK. Don't feel obligated to remain friends with someone just because of your history. You're constantly evolving and changing throughout life, and this means you'll have to move on and leave behind people who aren't evolving in the way you'd hope for in a friend. Odds are, you probably wouldn't be compatible with your high school boyfriend anymore, and the same goes for a former bestie. We all change, and our friends change in their own ways, too. No one expects you to keep dating the same guy for ten years if you don't mesh well anymore. The same concept applies to friends.

I know it may seem like it isn't a big deal to keep deadbeat friends around. Sure, she's not a bad bitch. Maybe she's not even someone you enjoy spending time with that much. But what's the harm of picking up when she calls or hanging out with her when you'd otherwise be kicking around alone? Just like every other aspect of your life, your friendships contribute directly to your overall confidence and success in the world. And what you might not realize is that maintaining relationships with people you're incompatible with actually takes a lot of energy. It's draining. If you make new, fabulous friends who are on your wavelength and understand you, they can help lift you up.

You're constantly evolving and changing throughout life, and this means you'll have to move on and leave behind people who aren't evolving in the way you'd hope for in a friend.

If you're unsure of a friend's place in your life, do the following exercise to assess a long-term friendship. Ask yourself, *If I met her today, would I make her my friend?* And then be brutally honest with yourself. Often enough, the answer is no, because you may not have anything in common with that person anymore, and the friendship only survives out of convenience or habit. If the answer is no, don't feel bad about it. When necessary, cut bitches loose. She'll probably be better off anyway.

GOOD FRIENDS GIVE TOUGH LOVE

You may realize you *would* be friends with a girl, but she's doing something that's bringing her down and threatening to bring you down with her. If you've decided you want to preserve this friendship because you really care about the person, and you know she has the potential to be a bad bitch with a little love and support, it's up to you to have a heart-to-heart with her. Sometimes people need tough love. Don't be mean or bitchy, but be honest.

If you had to carry your friend out of the club the previous night, let her know it's not cool. "Look, I'm talking to you because I actually care about you," you could say. "I want you to have the incredible life you deserve, but this kind of behavior isn't doing anything for you."

Sometimes it's really hard to talk to a friend about a subject you can tell is sensitive for her. But that's what friends are for. One of my old friends from Philly had a baby with a man she really loved, and then he left her for a younger woman. She was devastated, and it took her a long time to heal her heart. Now she's finally gotten back on top and learned to rock it as a single mom. Only every now and again, he'll come around again, sending her flowers or doing something nice for her. And she feels obligated to sleep with him, not as a way of trying to get back with him but almost as a way of saying thank you. "That's your daugh-ter's father," I say. "You don't have to sleep with him because he does something nice for you. You already did the nicest possible thing in the world for him. You gave him a beautiful daughter. That's more than enough."

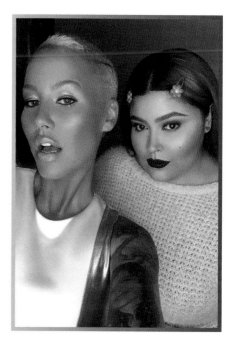
Besties

If your friend can tell that you're speak-ing out of genuine care for her, and she really cares about you, too, then she will appreciate your honesty. She'll listen to what you're say-ing and take your feelings and opinions into consideration. On the other hand, if she gets defensive and angry and makes it clear all she wants to do is the exact opposite of what you value, maybe she should be close with someone else instead. No judgment. Maybe you just want dif-ferent lifestyles, and that's OK.

As you grow up, you create your own way of living—in your case, a bad-bitch lifestyle. Not all of your friends have to come along with you, and you don't have to hold yourself back in order to stay with them. You just have to know when it's time to make some new friends and let the old ones go. At least you tried to help your friend, and maybe she'll even come around when she gets her act together and be grateful that you respected her enough to tell her the truth. If not, don't be afraid to move on.

Back in Philly, I had a friend for fifteen years. We were so close that I used to call him my brother. Maybe a year into when I started getting noticed, he put up a website advertising my appearances. My secu-

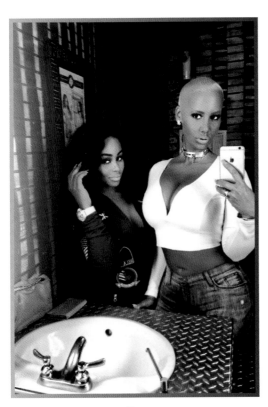

Bathroom selfie with my sis Chyna

rity came across it online and told me. I knew I had nothing to do with the site, and yet it was saying it represented me.

I called the number listed. "I wanted to know if you guys book Amber Rose," I said.

"Yes, we do," said the girl who answered.

"No, you don't, honey, because this is Amber Rose," I said. "Who are you?"

"We take care of your bookings," she said. I actually felt bad for her, because it was clear she'd been fed a whole pack of lies and had no idea what was going on.

"No, baby, you don't take care of my bookings," I said.

When I asked her who she worked for, she dropped my friend's name, and that hurt. I couldn't believe he'd done that to me. She told me that he'd been booking events for me, having the client wire the first half of the payment to his account. When I didn't show up, he never got the second half, but that didn't matter to him. He'd already gotten a fat payment for doing nothing. Meanwhile, he was hurting my reputation. I never talked to him again, I just saw that the site immediately went down, and I knew from the fact that he never called me to explain or defend himself that he'd been guilty. And we're talking about fifteen years of friendship, over in a day.

No matter how long you've known someone, you don't owe them shit if they're lying to you or treating you badly. You definitely can't have people like that in your world. They'll only bring you down.

Yes-People Are a No-No

Sure, sometimes we do need tough love just as much as our friends do. We can be blind. I definitely recommend listening to anything a real friend has to tell you. But never forget to take a step back and look at what you truly want. If friends do give you advice, it should be because they are looking out for your best interests, not because they're trying to tell you how to live. Those are two totally different things, and the distinction is very important, even when it comes to little things like your fashion choices. If your friend is constantly trash-talking you, like "Ugh, don't wear that. Don't do your hair like that," and your look is something you really love, then they've got to go. If they can't understand your chosen form of self-expression, or at least respect it, it's see-you-never. But if a friend is expressing concern about your well-being, then that's a different thing. And it can be a sign that she really cares about you.

There's nothing more dangerous than having nothing but "yes"-people around you. You *cannot* trust them. Maybe they're just going along with what they think you want, because they think it will make you like them, or maybe they have bad judgment. Either way, it's a problem. If you say you're going to do something that isn't good for you, like telling somebody off or spending money you don't really have on something you don't really need, they're the ones who egg you on. "Yeah, yeah, fucking do it," a yes-girl will say. When, really, that's the last thing you need to do, and a real friend would respectfully suggest that you stop a minute and think it through. You don't need yes-people in your life, because they're a part of the problem, not the solution.

Knowing you've trusted your intuition and done your best to stand up for yourself makes every difficult transition easier. Sometimes we're still going to face an outcome that's heartbreaking and hard, but it's so much easier to make peace with it if we've listened to ourselves, rather than caving in to peer pressure and feeling obligated to cater to other people's advice or feelings. This can be a really hard lesson to learn, especially when the people advising you are people you love and who you know love you, but it's an important part of growing up and becoming a bad bitch.

OK, now that we've covered what goes into maintaining a good, solid friendship, I'm going to go over the different types of friends every girl should have.

THE GAY BEST FRIEND

I'm very serious about this: every girl should have a gay best friend. There are so many reasons. Obviously, it's a stereotype that all gay boys know about fashion and makeup, but my gay friends do tend to give me some of the best inspiration and feedback on my look ever. And whatever my gay BFFs are talking to me about, they tend to be really honest and up-front. I think this has to do with how much courage it can take to realize you're gay and come out to your family and the world, even when there are still so many haters out there. Going through all of that can't help but build inner strength and confidence, and that's bound to make them into certified bad bitches. You don't want people tearing you down, but you also do want to have people around who will be real with you.

THE LIFE-OF-THE-PARTY FRIEND

Your party friends are a special category, and while your conversations often stay at surface level, they are still indispensable. Maybe they're not people you would tell all your personal business to, but they'll definitely show you a good time. They're always down to have fun. You absolutely need friends like that. I don't expect these friends to start a business with me or come

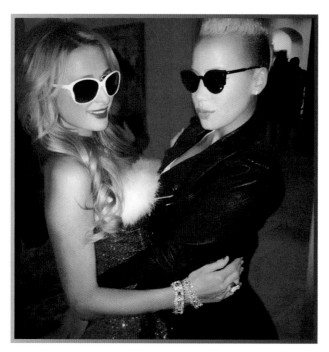

over and watch movies when I'm sick with the flu, but when I want to party hard, they are always up for an adventure, and they keep me laughing.

Fun with my bad bitch Paris

From my experience, it's a good idea always to have a couple of straight male friends who are like brothers to you. They can be invaluable for giving you advice and helping you to see the male perspective. And if you're going through a dry period on the dating front, they can be great for your self-esteem. Just being around a guy can make you feel more girlish and desirable, even if you wouldn't go there with him in a million years.

Just be clear on one thing: they will probably want to sleep with you, even if you make it known it's never going to happen. They might never tell you they want you, but that's how the male mind works. Men are just different. So don't get undressed in front of them, and always keep it in the friend zone. You may think I'm exaggerating, but in my experience, once the line even comes close to being crossed, there's no going back.

I had one male friend growing up, and I'd known him since kindergarten. He was like a brother to me. I had zero interest in him romantically. I just didn't think of him like that. When we were in high school, we'd go out to the club sometimes, and he'd come over to my place while I was getting ready. I was so relaxed with him that I changed clothes in front of him without even thinking about it. I mean, I had my underwear and bra on, so nothing was really showing, and he seemed cool with it, so I didn't think much of it. But then, two days later, he texted me: *Amber, the other day when you were getting undressed I realized how beautiful you were. I never really looked at you like that until then, but now I can't stop thinking about it.* He wasn't creepy about it or anything, but I couldn't even be his friend anymore. After almost twenty years of friendship, he threw it out the window because his feelings changed and mine didn't. So be mindful of your behavior. And don't be surprised if this

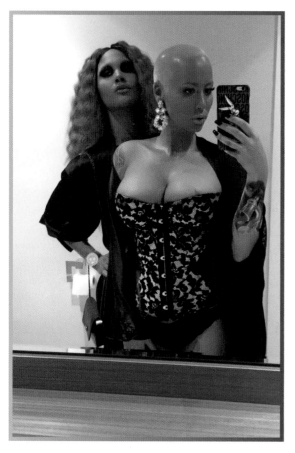

Muva and Dawta

happens to you, too. If he's a good friend, you might work through it. But sometimes you just can't.

If you're the one who wants to take it to the next level, really think about it first. If you just suddenly notice that he's cute, is that really worth potentially messing up a good friendship when there are plenty of fine men out there? On the other hand, if you realize he's the love of your life and you know that you guys already get along great as friends, maybe you could have an incredible roman-

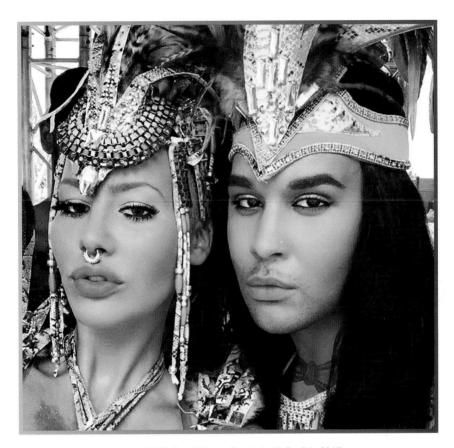

. At the Trinidad and Tobago Carnival with Benji in 2015

tic relationship. So, by all means, say something. Be very clear—with yourself and with him—that you're not interested in just a friendship anymore. If it's obvious he doesn't feel the same way, don't just hang around pretending to be his friend forever, hoping he'll fall in love with you someday. Have some self-respect, sister. If you can be cool staying in the friend zone, good, but if not, keep it moving.

While we're on the subject of platonic relationships with men, let me be perfectly clear about something very important: a bad bitch does not mix business and pleasure. So don't think for a second that the rumors about Nick and me being together are true. We do business together. Neither of us would ever go there, and you never should, either.

THE INNER CIRCLE

Let me tell you, when your personal business has a tendency to end up in the tabloids, you learn how to determine whom you can trust and whom you can't—fast. Go with your gut, and always err on the side of caution. Weigh out the pros and cons of every friendship. If someone's a fun girl but has a known tendency to run her mouth, it's best to keep her as a party friend or cut her out of your life completely.

Never rush trust, because only time can reveal someone's worthiness. There's no reason to confide in anyone who doesn't clearly have your back 100 percent. This is a very important rule. Let me tell you, just as with finding the right guy, there are millions of women out there who could potentially be your friend. Don't settle for anyone who's not going to up your game. If a girl's not treating you well, find a new friend who will.

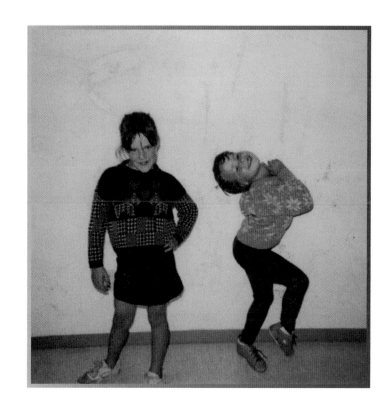

In Fort Drum, New York, around age five or six, with my childhood best friend Dawn. My mom had cut my hair to look like a punk witch . . . now you see where I get it from!

Once you have your inner circle in place, do unto your friends as you would want them to do unto you. Be extremely loyal. Let them know they're appreciated. And have fun with them. Life is meant to be enjoyed. That's the whole point of getting our bad bitch on in the first place, so we can all live the best lives possible.

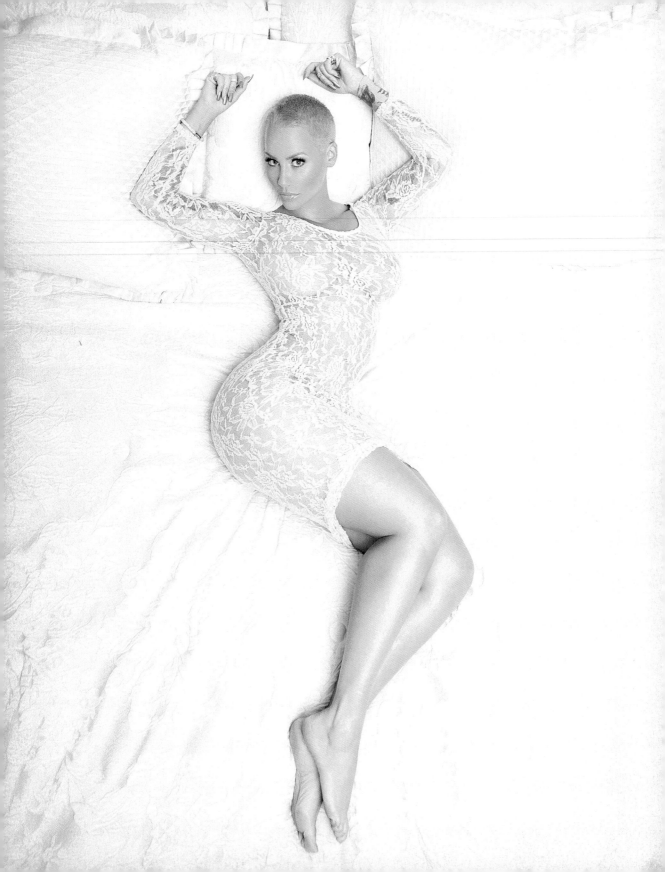

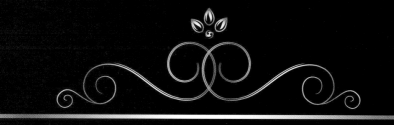

9
DATING

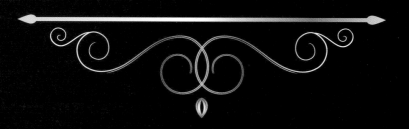

There's no denying that we ladies love everything that has to do with love, from flirtation and sex to marriage and babies. Though relationships can be emotional, they don't have to be painful, if you get smart. If anybody knows how men work, it's me. Let me tell you, this is a book of mistakes. I've made them all, but the good thing is I've learned from them.

You could also say I'm reminding you of the importance of priorities, ladies. I'm all for getting pleasure out of life, but it's really important to keep your eye on the prize and put yourself first. It's only now, after you've gotten yourself in check, that you're ready to mingle.

A GIRL CAN BE BOLD

I definitely think a girl can be bold when it comes to giving out her number, but she's got to do it with a little finesse. Go up to him, smile, and hand him your digits without a fuss. Then the ball is in his court. You don't have to look thirsty by texting him first. You don't have to stress yourself out, sitting around, wondering, *Should I text him? Is it too late? Is it too early?* Of course, this leaves you slightly vulnerable, because there's always a chance he won't hit you up. That's the worst thing he can do, though, and honestly, it's no big deal. If he's not interested, he's not interested. There truly is a guy out there for everyone. But if he does text you, don't text him back for ten minutes. You're busy, ladies.

If you really like a guy, I do think it can be cute to even go a little further and ask him out. Just don't be desperate or clingy about it. Be cool and confident, and he'll probably be intrigued enough to want to take you up on your offer and see what you're all about. In my experience, a casual approach is best. When you have a minute alone with him or get him on the phone, adopt a flirty, playful tone: "I want to take *you* on a date. I want to take you out to eat." Life and love don't have to be so serious all the time, especially when you're just getting to know someone. Guys like girls who are confident enough to enjoy themselves. They also like to be treated well, just like we do. Offering to do something for a guy you like can go far.

DATING LIKE A BAD BITCH

Going on a date is not going over to a guy's house and chilling with his friends while they drink beer and play video games. That comes later on,

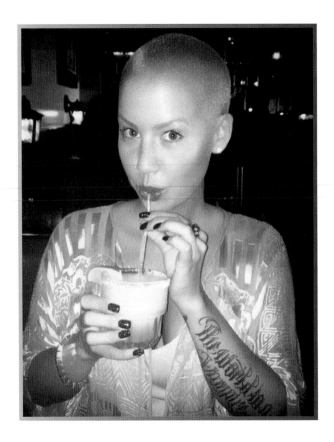

when you're in a relationship. Something to look forward to, right? An actual date is a restaurant, a movie, bowling—somewhere he takes you (or you take him) *without* a bedroom nearby. A great guy will want to show you his chivalry by opening doors, pulling out chairs, and being a true gentleman. Don't settle for a booty call unless that's all you really want it to be. If you want to date, be clear about your intentions, and all will unfold as it was meant to. Maybe you're worried a direct approach will scare him off. But this is the thing, right? When you first meet someone, you really have nothing to lose. If you tell him exactly what you want, you may get exactly what you want. Who cares what happens that early in a potential relationship? You're there to have fun, not to marry the first guy you see! If he doesn't respect you, better to know now and move on, rather than possibly fall for a guy who's not at all serious about you.

As Sexy as She Wants to Be

I know there are a lot of ideas out there about how sexy a girl should or shouldn't dress on her first date or how far she should or shouldn't go. I think she should feel free to dress as sexy as she wants to be. I don't think there's any limit; cleavage, legs out, that's all fine. Just remember, a guy will treat you the same way you dress, so keep that in mind as you're getting ready.

Be Honest

If the date isn't going the way you think it should, just be honest and tell him. If he says he's taking you to dinner and then he pulls into a McDonald's, you've got a right to say something. If he's on his phone the whole time, say something like, "I came out on a date with

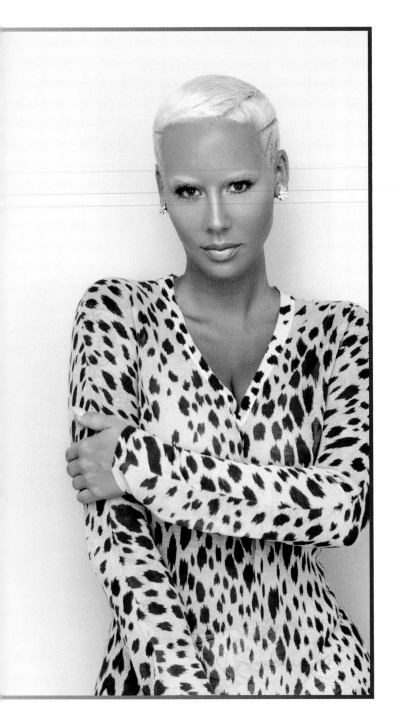

you, and you're constantly on the phone. I think it's rude. I came here for you." There's nothing wrong with speaking up. If you don't, and he thinks you're happy with things as they are, then you're never going to get what you want. And if you're already letting him take advantage of your kindness, there's trouble ahead. Or maybe you're afraid to speak up because you worry he might snap back. But if that's who he is, you need to see it on the first date, because then you'll know he's an asshole, and you've got to—you guessed it—keep it moving. Let me tell you something. If you and this guy end up falling in love, you may think that's enough to be happy. But love's not the only important component of a relationship. Respect is a huge part of dating, too, and if he's disrespecting you early on, which is when people are supposedly on good behavior, then what's he going to be like when you're having a fight? And I hope it goes without saying that if he ever raises more than his voice at you—or even suggests that he might be thinking about hurting you—you're out of there. It's always better to get out at the first sign of hostility. You deserve to be safe. You never know—you could say something, and it could actually make him rethink his behavior enough that you want to see him again.

For example, when I was maybe seventeen and living in Philly, this guy took me out to eat, and he was really mean to the waitress. I did not hesitate to speak my mind.

"What the fuck is your problem, dude?" I said. "My mom raised me on a waitress's salary. She was a waitress for thirty years, so you treating her like that makes me feel like you would treat my mother like that if you didn't know it was my mom." I was pissed, like I was ready to walk out of there.

But he made it right. "I'm so sorry," he said. "I didn't think about it that way."

"Well, you need to look at everybody with the idea that she's someone's mother, sister, daughter. Think about your own family members and how you'd want them to be treated before you treat people badly. Maybe our waitress is busy. Maybe somebody called out sick today, and she's trying to take care of everybody in here by herself, so she can make money to take care of her baby or whatever the case may be."

"You're absolutely right," he said. I could tell he was being sincere.

When the waitress came back to take our order, he was on his best behavior, and he tipped her very well that night. I liked him enough to go out with him several times, and he never disrespected a waitress again. In the end, we weren't a good fit, but at least I gave it a chance. It can feel really good to help someone have a different perspective, instead of just assuming he's a jerk. Often, he'll turn out to be a decent person if you give him the opportunity to be. This guy did. Even if he hadn't, at least I would have known I'd stood up for myself and my mom. That's why a bad bitch speaks her mind.

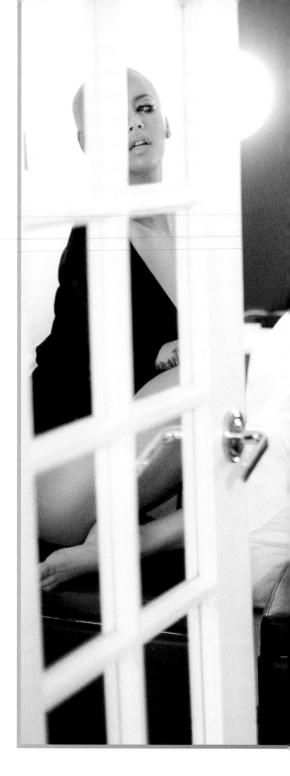

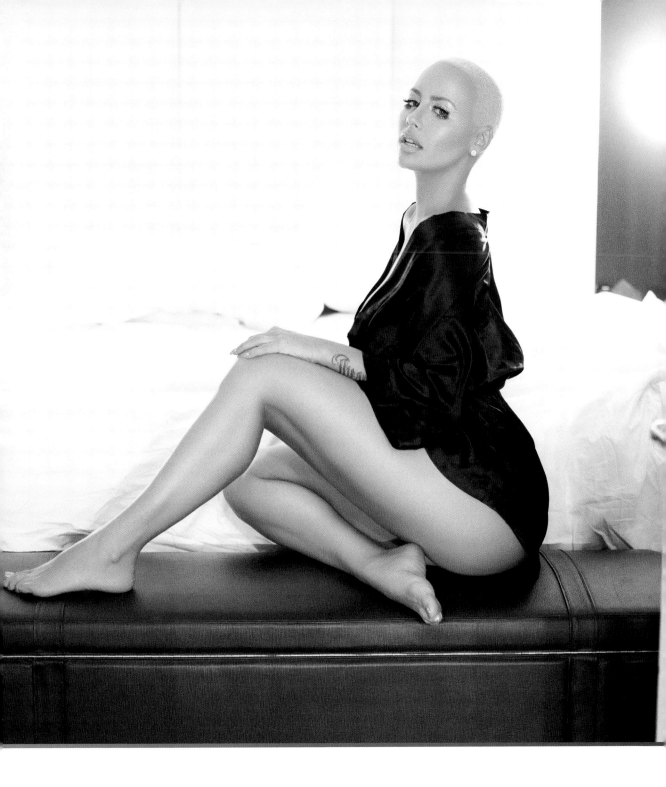

HOW TO BE A BAD BITCH

Other bad behaviors can't necessarily be made right, though. There are serious warning signs, ladies. If a guy puts you down in any way, don't stand for it. If he critiques your outfit, your hair, your makeup, or anything else you have going on that day or if he's critical of your lifestyle or your family, deal breaker. That's just the beginning of a fucking nightmare. Sure, if you ask him for his opinion and he tells you—nicely—that he's not into your look or something else in your life, it could maybe still work out. And if he's just plain rude, give him the opportunity to make it right—by killing him with kindness. A bad bitch always takes the high road. Voicing your feelings with straightforward grace is always the best way to go. Try your hardest not to go from zero to a hundred or turn it into an argument. If he's just an asshole, he's not worth it. And if he's a nice enough guy that you end up dating, you'll have plenty of real fights about serious stuff, so just let this one go. Learning how to recognize negativity is a good lesson when going forward with a relationship. Not only will it help you to determine what's unacceptable behavior from him, but it will also frame how you approach your man.

A lot of girls, for better or worse, think they know who their guys should be—from their interests to their humor to their wardrobes. They are constantly trying to remake their boyfriends, and as far as I'm concerned, that's just trouble. If you meet a guy and he's been drinking every single night, don't think that when you get into a relationship or get married, he's suddenly going to stop. People don't work that way. If you're not a fan of his clothing style and he ends up being your boyfriend, you can go out and buy him something you'd like him to wear. But if he isn't responsive to that, that's OK. That's when you have to decide to like him for who he is or keep it moving. I, personally, don't ever try to change anyone. It seems disrespectful to me. Why create problems for yourself?

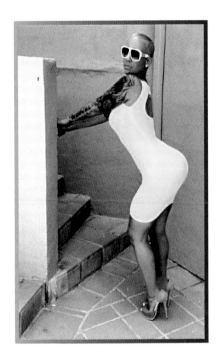

A First Date Is Not the Third Degree

Obviously, if you like a guy, you're going to want to get some information about him, because you're curious to know what he's all about. Does he want to have kids? Has he ever been in a serious relationship before? Has he ever lived with someone? Has he ever been married? All in good time, ladies. First-date questions should be light, breezy, and fun. Enjoy yourself. See if you like his company. So many women get so nervous about first dates, but that's exactly what it is: a first! You have no idea

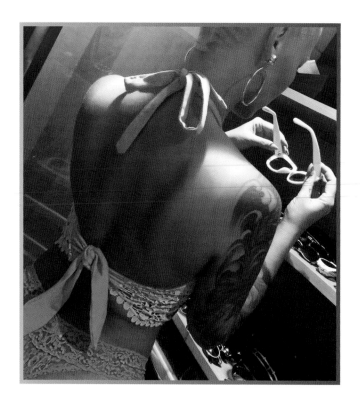

if you two will even get along, so there's nothing to worry about.

Then, if you have a second date, you can start to dig a little deeper. Maybe you start to ask him about his family. And try to get a sense—without asking for his tax returns—of how he's doing professionally and where he hopes to be headed in life. How quickly you get serious after that depends on where you are in life and what you're looking for. If you're just out of school and want to have fun, you might keep it casual for a while. If you're in your thirties and want to have children, time is of the essence, and if you make it to a third date, you'll probably want to find out where he's at in his life. You can ask questions more along the lines of "Do you like kids?" By this point, you know you've got some chemistry, so it's OK to get a little more serious and see if there's real potential. I know some people might think this is too soon. But hell, as far as I'm concerned, you should feel it's your right to bring it up on the *first* date. No, I don't mean making some kind of big declaration like "By this time next year, I'd like to be pregnant, and I'm wondering if you'll be my baby daddy." You definitely don't want to say anything that will put too much pressure on him—or you. But if you're on a date with someone because you think he could be a potential partner, and not because you just want to hook up with him, then I definitely think it's better to know sooner rather than later if he's a good fit or not. You don't want to fall for him and then realize it's not going to work out because you want totally different things from life. This is especially true if you're already a mom. Then you should definitely mention it on the first date. Your kid is too important to even mess with the possibility of ending up with a guy who doesn't absolutely love children and feel confident that he wants them in his life.

KNOW YOUR DEAL BREAKERS

I think all of us want love, but for many of us, our desires take very different forms. Some women want mad physical chemistry. Some want to be with a man who's just as ambitious as they are, so they won't have to feel guilty about putting their careers first. Some want to be with a man who can carry his own financially, because they work hard and they don't need someone draining off their finances or doing anything less than carrying at least half of the expenses in the relationship. Now, that doesn't mean you should measure everything in dollar signs.

One of the coolest dates I've ever been on was an early-morning hike with a guy who was encouraging me to keep climbing through the pain (it's harder than it looks!) and being supportive on what turned out to be a really difficult trail. Afterward, we went out to eat, and we had dirt and sand all over us, and we didn't even care. We were feeling so good because of what we'd done. That's what really brought us together. Our newfound bond and accomplishment was what made the date great.

Life and love don't have to be so serious all the time, especially when you're just getting to know someone.

A good date can be really sweet, even if it doesn't end up being a love connection. And who knows? Even if it doesn't work out, you could have made a new friend. A bad date, well, that's a different story. At least you know you'll have a good story for later. I'm a big believer in good manners, but if a guy is rude or demeaning, it's always appropriate to get up and leave. The whole point of being a bad bitch is to live your life to the fullest and be happy. It doesn't have to be a whole big dramatic moment where you throw a drink in his face. Keep it classy, grab your things, and go. You'll be glad you did.

When I was eighteen, this guy took me to the movies. Theaters had just started putting in those armrests that go up, so you can snuggle with each other. I thought the guy was cute, so I lifted the armrest and started to get close to him. "Whoa, whoa, whoa, whoa," he said, pulling away. I couldn't believe what I was seeing as he smoothed down his shirt so it wouldn't get wrinkled, and then he looked at me expectantly. "OK, now it's OK," he whispered. He was more concerned about his shirt getting wrinkled than about being next to me. That might not sound like that big a deal, but it really hurt my feelings. Why had he even asked me out if he didn't want to be near me? I was so turned off that I couldn't wait to leave, and I never spoke to him again. He was clearly *not* for me. Now I can look back and laugh, but back then I was really unhappy about that date.

I'm sure you have your share of war stories from the dating front lines, whether you're in a happy relationship or still looking for that special someone. No matter what happens out there, just be sure to respect yourself and try to have as much fun as possible, and eventually, you'll meet the one. And then, it's relationship time.

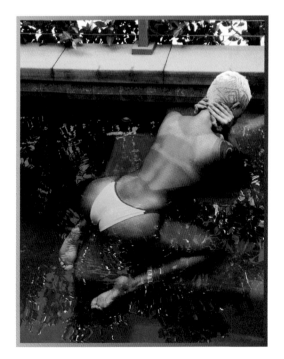

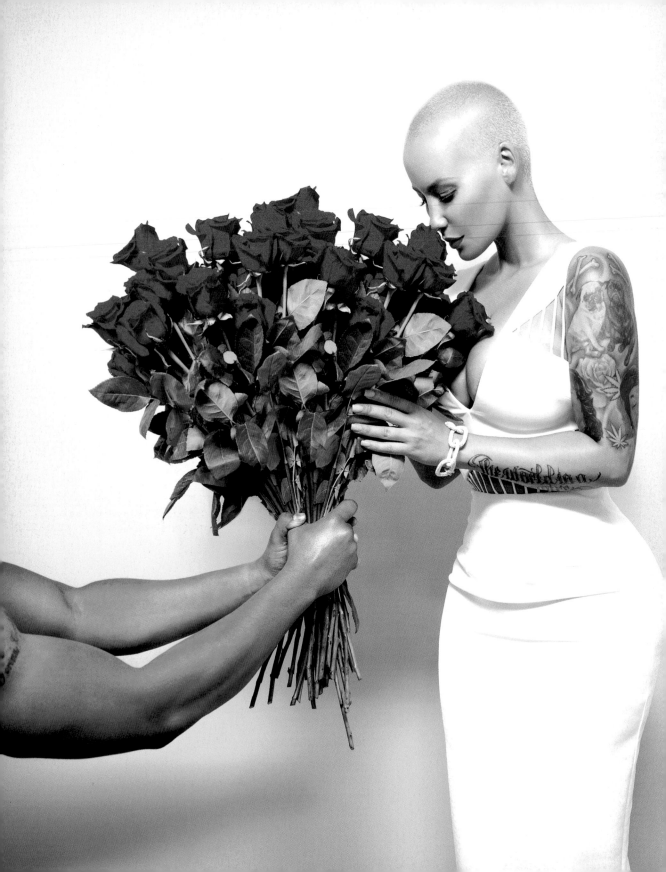

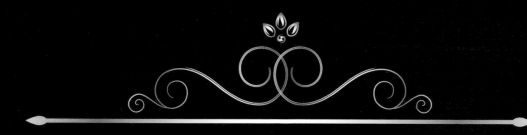

10

RELATIONSHIPS

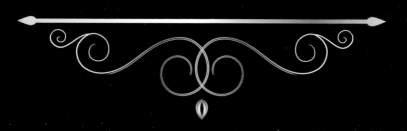

Too often, I think women have this idea that if they want a relationship, they have to follow certain rules. The truth is, you should always take risks, because you never know what's going to happen. If you're on a first date and you're wondering if you should make the first move or invite him in, never forget that it's your call. Guys are always ready and willing to come in. So it's really your decision. Maybe you're thinking, *Fuck it, I want him to come in. I want to make out with him or snuggle with him or sleep with him.* Whatever you want to do, you should do it. You should take the initiative to say, "Do you want to come in? Do you want to hang out for a while?" I don't think there's anything wrong with that. And nine times out of ten, the guy's not going to say no.

There are a ton of supposed rules out there about how far girls should be willing to go on dates, especially if they want the guy to be their boyfriend. As far as I'm concerned, if you want to have sex on the first night, that's your business. You don't have to feel bad about it, and it doesn't automatically mean he won't be your boyfriend. You could move toward a relationship after that and if you do end up together, it doesn't matter when the first time was anyhow. But if you're going to sleep with him on the first night, you should be cool with the fact that he might not call you again. Then, no matter what happens, you can say to yourself, *Fuck it. I had a good time. I did what I wanted to do. I lived my life.*

Oops

Sometimes it's easy to let go and lose your cool, especially early on in a relationship. There isn't much to lose yet. Maybe you slept with him and he never called you again, so you drunk-dialed him or texted him a piece of your mind in a fit of passion. Maybe you were just a little clingy or annoying, which is a definite bad-bitch no-no. But we've *all* lost it, at one point or another. Drunk-dialing, or any inappropriate behavior of that nature, should definitely be followed up with some kind of note. But keep your tone very light—maybe even make fun of yourself by sending him a hungover smiley-face emoticon or writing something like "Ha ha, I was so drunk last night. No more drinks for me for a while." Don't necessarily feel like you have to turn it into a serious apology. Keep the conversation casual, and then move it to a new topic. And don't bring it up again. There's nothing cooler than a girl who doesn't take herself so seriously. And, as always, if he's not an understanding guy, better to know sooner rather than later.

WHAT GUYS LIKE

Every guy has slightly different tastes, sure. But more often than not, guys are looking for pretty much the same thing in a woman. Knowing their quirks gives you the upper hand. Here are five things guys like:

1 Girls who can hang with the guys—and, sad but true—play video games—but who can still be very feminine.

2 Girls who don't get jealous or weird.

3 Girls who have good manners and aren't always burping and cussing like a guy.

4 Girls who are put together but not afraid to get messy in the bedroom.

5 Girls who aren't afraid to treat them on a date or give a little gift.

Maybe the guy is the one who messes up. He stands you up and claims he had to work late . . . two days later. Or he gets too drunk and you have to take care of him all night. Or he's the one who drunk-dials you. Though it's never fun when a guy fucks up, you need to realize everyone makes mistakes. Everyone fucks up, drunk-dials, or is late sometimes. Everyone says something he didn't mean or loses his cool once in a while. Who knows? Maybe he had a family emergency, and he didn't feel comfortable opening up to you about it yet. Try to give him the benefit of the doubt and not be too bitchy over one screw-up. As long as it's not an ongoing pattern of flaky or unsavory behavior, you should try to forgive and forget, because you would want the same in return.

If a guy is late or doesn't call, many women automatically jump to the conclusion that he's doing something he's not supposed to be doing—maybe with another woman—and instantly cop an attitude. But you don't know what happened. Even if it is a situation where you find out he's not being as respectful of you and your time as he should be, there's definitely something to be said for the classy approach. Sometimes it's better to wait a few hours and then call him with a concerned tone of voice. "Damn, babe, you were supposed to call me two hours ago. Is everything OK?" Instead of telling him off, try being more interested in what happened and why he didn't end up doing what he was supposed to do. If something did happen to waylay him, you won't seem like a total bitch. And even if he was just goofing off with his friends, as long as you let him know he needs to be respectful of your time, having a positive attitude can go far. If you're always the bigger person, the majority of the time, he'll want to be around you more than anybody else. As long as you're not a doormat, being nice is the best approach.

DON'T PRETEND

While it's OK to show him you like him, if you feel like you're not getting the same kind of consideration in return, you've got to move on. That goes for how independent he's comfortable with you being, too. In my

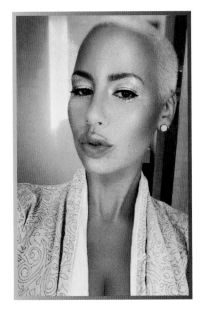

experience, most guys like a woman who's got her own life and isn't too clingy, and that works well for me. But some men want a woman who's completely submissive.

I was getting to know this guy, and we decided I should visit his hometown so we could get to know each other better. While I was making my travel plans, he got mad that I rented my own car instead of asking him if I could borrow his. I was polite, but basically my attitude was *I've got my own money, and I barely know you, so I'd feel more comfortable taking care of myself.* He could not get over it. I'd never been around a guy who would get angry about something that had absolutely nothing to do with him, except for the fact that he didn't get to have all of the power in the situation. For me, that kind of controlling streak outweighed the other aspects of his personality that I liked, and I knew he wasn't the one for me. Of course, if you're the type of girl who gets off on being submissive, you've got to do what makes you happy. Just don't pretend it's OK if it's not.

SHOW THEM WHO YOU REALLY ARE

It's tempting to be overaccommodating and pretend to be "flawless" at the beginning of a relationship. At that stage, we would often prefer to please the other person, rather than show them who we really are. Though we may want to bury our shortcomings, ladies, the beginning of a relationship is the perfect moment to be very honest. I know, I know, I've heard it before. "It's not like I'm *lying* to him. I'm just keeping him happy." And I get it. I do. But there's a danger in piling it on. "Baby, you want breakfast? I'm going to cook you dinner. Let me rub your back and iron your laundry. This is just who I am. I'll be like this forever." Inevitably, he'll find out that you're not really that girl, and you'll have to start from scratch.

If he doesn't love who you truly are, it's better to know now. When you really like someone, be brutally honest about yourself from the door. If you're not the best cook, you don't want to have kids, you're not into whatever the hell he's into, don't lie about it. Be as honest as possible about who you are and what you want out of life and a relationship. That way, if the two of you do fall in love, he knows what he's in for from the beginning.

Let a man be a man. Even though you're capable of moving your living-room furniture around by yourself, ask for help, because men like to feel needed. That doesn't make you any less of a strong woman. At the same time, even if you find a man who can take care of you, don't ever stop being able to do for yourself. I used to let one of my exes discourage me from pursuing my own career interests, and looking back, I really regret that. Now that I've got my career up and running, I'll never sideline it for anyone again.

And don't ever give up your friends for a guy. For one thing, they've had your back since long before you knew him, and they deserve to be treated better than that. Also, many romantic relationships we think will last forever don't, or at least they have rough patches along the way, and you're going to need your ladies then. Honor them by maintaining those bonds, even when you've got a new man in your life.

GET OVER IT OR MOVE ON

There's that moment, early on in a relationship, when you sit down with your new man and you both come clean about your histories—your exes, your "number," your pitfalls, and your childhoods. This is a serious conversation, and you should only have it when you're ready. I don't, however, think you should ask how many sexual partners he's had, because it's irrelevant—not something you really need to know—and it could end up making you mad or haunting you once you really love him. You may disagree with this because you feel honesty is important at the beginning of a relationship, and I agree with you on that point. But I truly don't believe it's your business to know every detail of his past. That was before he met you. People grow and change, and if you like him enough to let him into your life, he deserves the chance

Though we may want to bury our shortcomings, ladies, the beginning of a relationship is the perfect moment to be very honest.

to show you who he is now, based on his current behavior, not having to live down who he used to be. If you do press him for details, however, know that when he tells you the truth, it's up to you to sit down and really think about whether you're willing to live with his past, because you can never bring it up again. If you like a guy but hate his past, really think about it. If he slept with a girl you don't like, is it a deal breaker? Does his past truly make your relationship impossible? If so, move on. If it's something you feel you can handle, you have to accept it and get on with life. A lot of girls have a really hard time with this, but you have to remember that the past is truly just history, not a guiding force of the future. It's up to you to

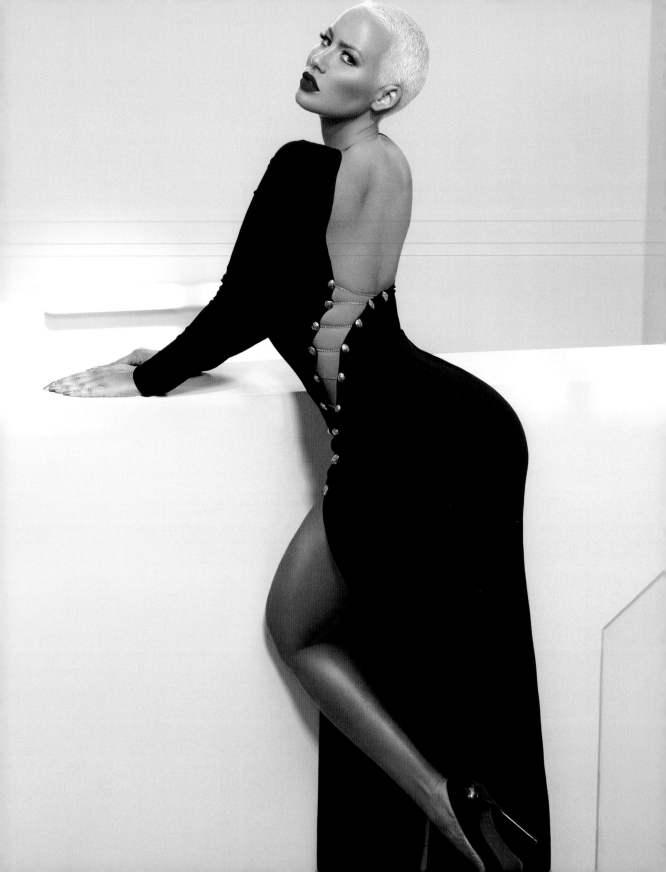

really be honest with yourself about what you can tolerate and what you can't. If you can't tolerate something, don't pretend you can, because you're not going to be happy. And as a result, he's not going to be happy. Trying in vain to "keep the peace" when you're actually upset about something always backfires eventually.

If you slept with one of his friends before you ever knew him, it's better to come clean about it of your own volition. You never want to go somewhere with your boyfriend, only to run into some guy from your past that your boyfriend doesn't know about. That secret will build and build and eventually manifest itself into burdensome anxiety. You've just got to lay down the facts: "Look, it was way before I ever met you. It happened, but now I've found you, and that's all that matters." And then, when you do run into that guy (which you inevitably will), you don't have to worry about anything. You never want the other guy to out you in front of your boyfriend, because that's the worst thing that could happen.

PEOPLE CHEAT, PERIOD

The sad truth is that love breeds denial on both sides. Both men and women often have a difficult time admitting they're not being fulfilled by their relationship, and rather than speak up about what they're feeling and what kinds of positive changes they'd like to see, they're often tempted to act out by cheating.

When the truth of someone's actions is finally unveiled, reality sinks in, and you eventually realize that you knew the whole time. You knew he wasn't happy. You knew he was cheating. You just didn't want to admit it.

As uncomfortable as it can be, the best thing you can do is be as honest as possible, as soon as possible. Try not to take his unhappiness too personally, even though it can be really painful to have him suddenly shut you out. If you really care about him, you want him to be happy, right? Try to make that the goal, rather than having an agenda about changing his behavior in a particular way.

When you talk to him about the state of your relationship, be very upfront, but be caring, too. Try saying something like "Look, I don't know what we should do right now, but we used to be friends, and you feel really far away from me right now. Maybe let's try for that closeness we used to have. Let's set up a date every week and start over by getting to know each other again. Because I love you, and I want to be with you, but all of this arguing is creating space between us. I don't want you to stay away from me, and I don't want to stay away from you, so we've got to find a way to come back together."

Maybe he'll come right out and admit he's not happy. Maybe he won't. Try not to point the finger at him—unless he's doing something really disrespectful that needs to be confronted—because if you do, you risk pushing him away farther. If he seems willing to work on things, too, try to show your appreciation for this effort and give it some time. Maybe your relationship can be salvaged. Maybe it's too far gone, and it can't be. But the earlier you speak up and the more care you show him, the more likely it will work out. Even though it's scary, sometimes showing some vulnerability, rather than anger, can go far. Send him flowers at work to show you still care, even though you guys are going through a rough patch. Do something nice for him, just because.

Sometimes showing some vulnerability, rather than anger, can go far.

In general, I think women are often more patient, compassionate, and loving than men, so it's up to us to set the tone in the relationship. If you're always trying to do the right thing and be kind, he'll remember that and appreciate you for it. Of course, if his behavior doesn't change or gets worse, you might have to consider ending it. If you want a deeper connection, better communication, more passion, you might have to find it elsewhere. Have the class to break up with him before you look outside the relationship for what you're not getting. If he doesn't have the integrity to do this, too, and you find out he's cheating on you, I know it hurts, but try to be as clear-headed as possible when you assess the situation and decide what to do next. You knew he wasn't happy. Now you have proof.

Men cheat, period. Maybe he hasn't cheated on you yet, but there will come a time when most men do seek fulfillment outside the relationship, whether it's with work, the gym, or another woman. Unfortunately, it's often with another woman, as an estimated twenty-five to seventy percent of married men cheat. It seems to be getting worse, too. Social media killed relationships forever, because a guy, especially a good-looking guy, can hit up a girl on Twitter or Instagram or Tinder, and it's on. Beautiful women are a dime a dozen, and many are easily accessible. It makes it so easy for men to just go out and do whatever. However, if you're really present in your relationship and you address any problems you two might be having as soon as possible, rather than staying in denial, maybe you can check his dissatisfaction before he acts on it.

Women cheat, too, and using the fact that men do it as an excuse for your own shady behavior is bullshit. Do you really want to be in that kind of relationship? If you're committed to him, put the time and energy into trying to save what you've got. If you're really tempted to forge a connection with another man—whether it's emotional, mental, or physical—have the decency to wait until you're single. You can't control how the men in your life will behave, but you can at least be responsible in your own actions.

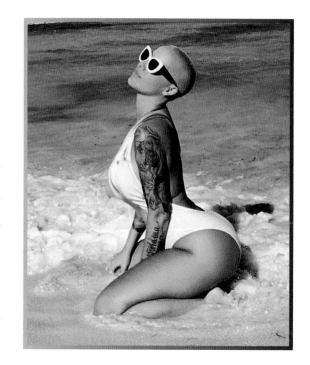

When you find out he's been unfaithful, you have to either forgive and forget or let him go and deal with the heartbreak. It's either one or the other. You can't stay with him after he cheated and then constantly throw it in his face. If you stay with him, you have to really forgive him, so you can move on as a couple.

When men cheat or they seriously fuck up, ignore the hell out of them. Don't answer their text messages. Don't answer their phone calls, until you feel like you've got them exactly where you want them. If you're too available, they know they still have you, and they're going to continue to do what they want to do. This may seem petty, but it's not about hurting his feelings just because he hurt yours. It's about sending him a message. Even though he may have disrespected you and your relationship, you

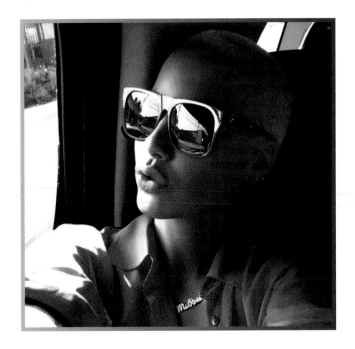

are still worthy of respect, and his actions have consequences. Maybe you are in the process of forgiving him and moving on with your relationship, but that takes time. Allowing a betrayal to happen and then instantly letting it blow over is going to send the message that his behavior wasn't that serious, and he'll be more tempted to do it again. If you ignore him, and he really realizes there's a good possibility he's lost you, that's when he's going to come around. If he doesn't, then it wasn't meant to be. Trying to persuade him to come back isn't going to work anyhow. Have some pride, ladies.

I do believe it's possible for there to be a scenario where the man—or the woman—cheats and there's genuine forgiveness and the relationship can get back to a happy place. Absolutely. I've seen it happen. I don't necessarily think it'll ever be the same, but I do believe in enduring love, for sure. I truly feel that if a man's dissatisfaction with your relationship has caused him to stray before you've had the chance to fix things, but he still really cares about you, he'll do everything in his power to hide his infidelities from you. If he's realized he was in the wrong and he knows he doesn't want to be with the other woman but he confesses to you just to clear his conscience, it will only be painful for you. I know you may think you absolutely need to know the truth, and I can see your point. But if it was just temporary insanity on his part, maybe it's better not to know. What you don't know won't hurt you. And what you do know can make it impossible for you to forgive him and rebuild your relationship. Once a man starts getting sloppy and he's getting phone calls and text messages and you're walking in and catching him, that's when he really doesn't give a fuck about you anymore. And you should really think twice about taking him back after this kind of behavior, not just because of the infidelity but because of the disrespect. I do believe men can be attracted to other women and make mistakes while still being in love with their wives and partners. But if he doesn't care enough about you to avoid rubbing it in your face, then that's a problem. If he really does care about you, he will protect your heart, even if he did something he now regrets.

R-E-S-P-E-C-T

Sometimes women are too worried about saving the relationship, when they should be more concerned with making sure the relationship is worth saving. If it's really not working, better to end it, so you can heal your

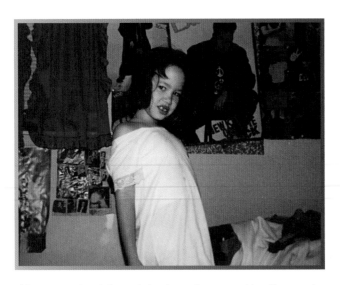

After my parents got divorced when I was six, we moved in with my aunt Ava. Here I am in my cousin's room, posing once again, this time with New Kids on the Block.

broken heart and move on. Even if there are kids involved, I think it's better for kids to go through a divorce than to constantly see their parents fighting and unhappy. Also, it can be better for the kids to have a really cool stepmom and stepdad, and maybe even some half brothers and half sisters, than to grow up in a house ruled by unhappiness. My parents got divorced when I was six, and I loved my stepdad and my stepmom and half brothers, and I'm so grateful for all of the family I have.

STAY STRONG

No matter what kind of circumstances you're living under, you really just have to know yourself. If you're genuinely happy with yourself, you won't let a man treat you badly or disrespect you. If he did cheat and you're both committed to rebuilding the relationship, that means you both have to be fully committed and willing to work on getting back to a good place. Then he can show his respect for you by doing the work.

Sometimes people actually can change for the good. There is nothing wrong with getting back with a person who's willing to make an effort to do better. This is another scenario where you have to trust your gut, though. It's easy enough for a man to say he's going to alter his behavior when he's afraid of losing you, but if he doesn't make any real effort, then you have to take a stand and go.

Sometimes women are too worried about saving the relationship, when they should be more concerned with making sure the relationship is worth saving.

Even if you're blissfully in love with a man who loves you back just as much and your relationship is strong and rewarding, never fully give your entire life and self to a man. Maintain some level of control, make your own decisions, and don't let a man manipulate you into doing things you don't want to do. It will make for a healthier relationship, and if the relationship ends, you'll be in a better place to start rebuilding. A bad bitch keeps some things for herself to feed her soul—just in case it doesn't work out. No woman should ever live in constant fear of losing something she feels she has, but at the same time, she should live with her eyes open. She should notice when things are going awry. It doesn't help that many men have these fucking egos and this fucking pride. They love a strong woman,

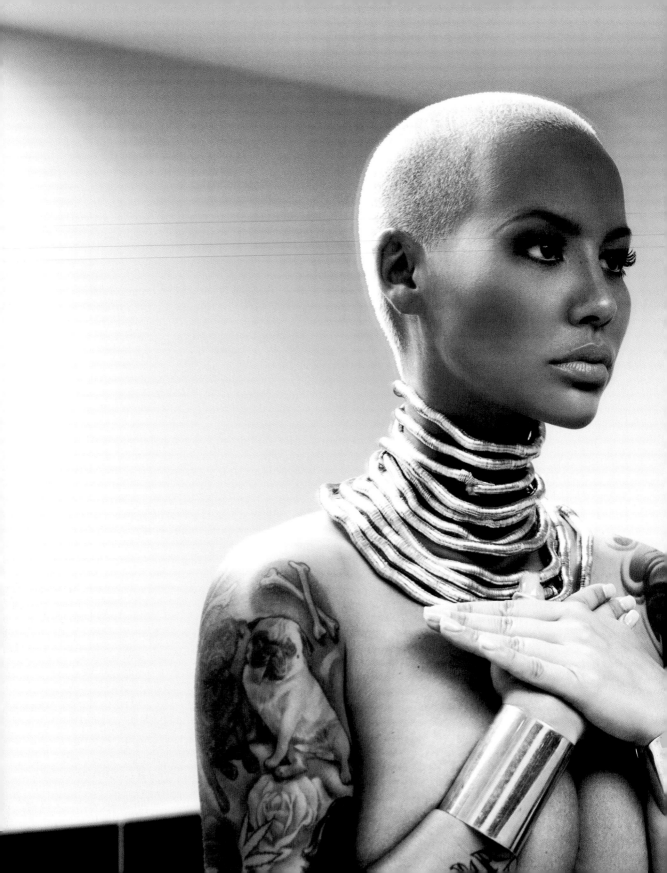

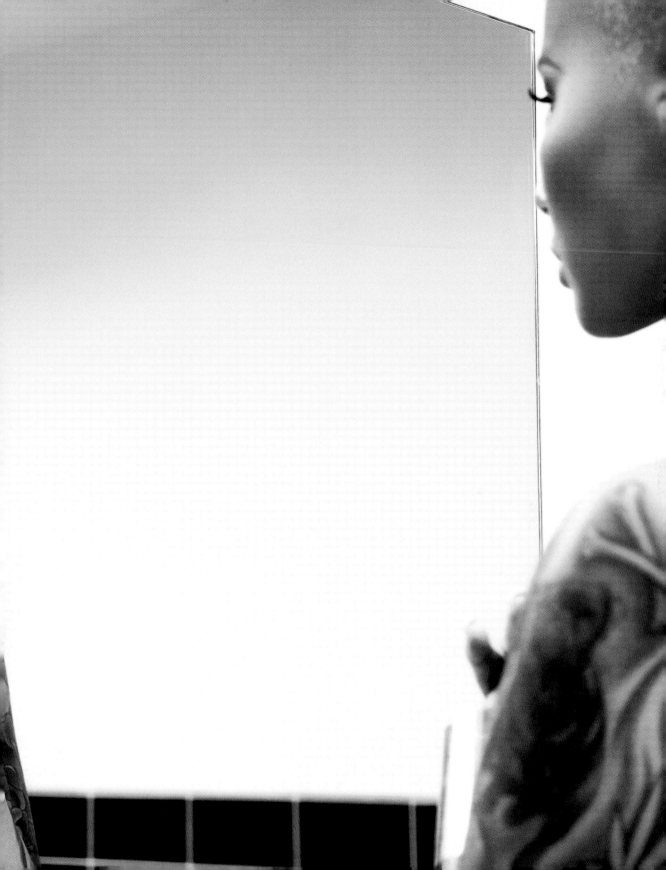

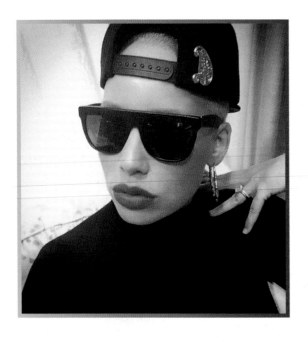

but then, once they get you, they've got to dumb you down and keep you in the house so no one else can look at you. Many men are super insecure. They see how good you are, and deep down, they're afraid of losing you.

I've given away too much of my power in every relationship I've ever had. I've always had a lot of great ideas I didn't do anything about, because I let my significant other belittle me or tell me I shouldn't go after them. Instead of supporting me and motivating me to do better in life, some men I've supposedly loved didn't want me to pursue my dreams, because they would inconvenience our relationship or make them insecure in their own accomplishments. Never again. I hope you ladies won't let it happen to you, either.

In the end, as hard as it can be, it's up to us to step away when necessary. We've just got to do it for ourselves. Life is short, and if I don't go for my goals, I'm going to regret it forever. That's how I live, day by day. Of course, there are men out there who will support you, love you, and encourage you to be who you are—but until you find that man, you've gotta keep looking.

SIDE PIECES

I know some girls will say, well, if men are going to cheat, then why shouldn't we keep someone on the side, too? I can see their point. But I don't see this kind of attitude leading anywhere good. I really believe you reap what you sow. I know guys can be really manipulative, but they have feelings, too, and they will be just as hurt if they find out you cheated as you were when their lies surfaced. Also, if I'm expecting my man to be faithful and devoted, except for when he makes a mistake and opts to right his behavior, then I believe he deserves the same from me. I know we've said that men usually cheat because they're unhappy in a relationship, and sure, women can be unhappy with their men, too. I'm just encouraging you to talk about your feelings and try to work things out, rather than stepping out on the side. I think the way men are wired, they're less likely to talk first, act later, but we have the opportunity to set a higher standard with our own behavior and to create better relationships with the men in our lives. Always aim to be the better person in life. That way, even if he does cheat and it doesn't work out, you'll know you gave your all to your relationship.

In the beginning, there is nothing wrong with casually dating multiple people to figure out who you belong with. But when you are in a relationship, you should give him the exact same respect you're craving, even if men don't always give us the respect we want and deserve. Stooping to the level of the worst man doesn't help.

There's a saying that the best way to get over someone is to get under someone else. Not to say that you need to run out and sleep with another guy, especially if you're still heartbroken and vulnerable, but it can be really healing to have someone in your life who makes you feel pretty again. It's nice to find someone who just makes you feel good, who you can hang out with, and make out with, and possibly have sex with, if you're ready. This person isn't your next boyfriend, he's just fun. There's nothing wrong with that. When he wants to come over and watch a movie just because he'd like to see you, or he gives you flowers or a gift, or

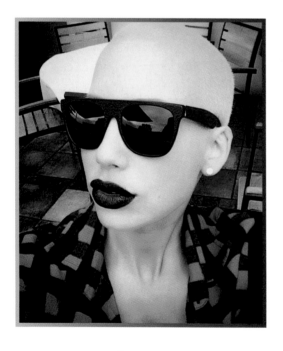

he calls you just to tell you that you're beautiful, it will remind you of all the value you've possessed this whole time, which the person who hurt you made you forget temporarily. Such little kindnesses really do help. After going through a breakup, especially with a man who's been extremely disrespectful and hurtful, it's nice to have a guy around who makes you feel special again. My mom has been single for six years, and I tell her all the time, "Ma, you need a rebound. You need to have a good time." If it's good enough for my mom, it's good enough for all of us.

Just remember, a rebound is a very specific type of relationship. The whole point is that it's not meant to be serious. You need time to heal and focus on yourself, and you don't want to get into a new relationship before you're ready. When you're vulnerable, you don't always have the best judgment, and you could end up picking another asshole. Better to spend a little time in a stress-free situation and wait to start mingling again until you're ready. Not that your rebound can't turn into more. But you shouldn't even be thinking about that yet. Just do you. Focus on getting back

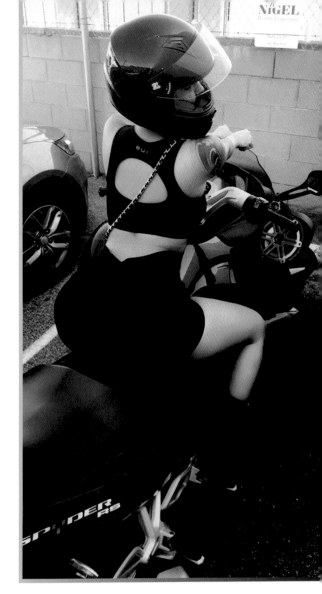

to the place where you can honestly think, *I'm a bad bitch. I'm a beautiful woman. I deserve to be happy. When I do have another guy in my life, I'm going to make sure he treats me well.*

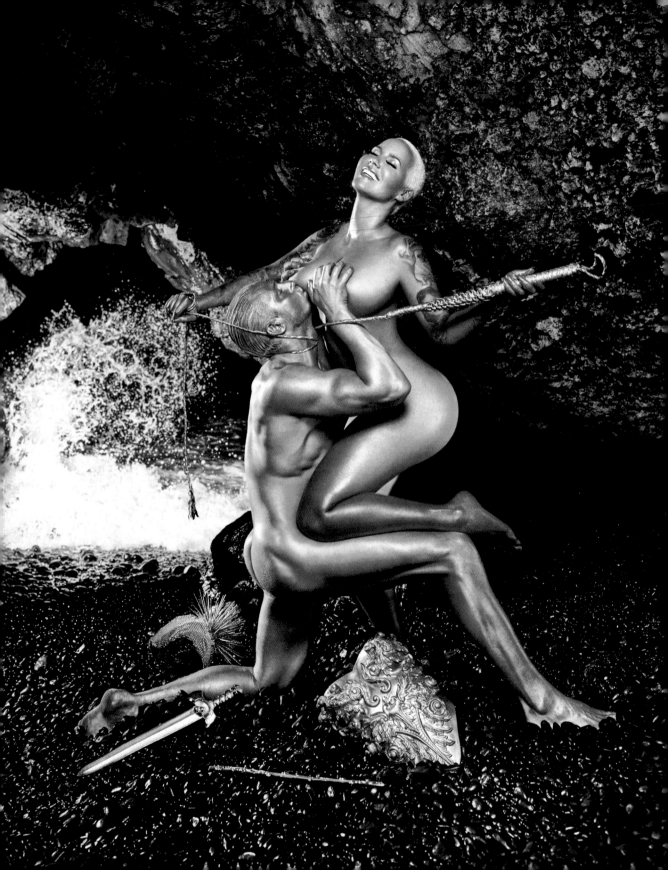

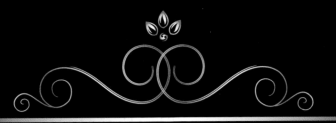

11
SEX

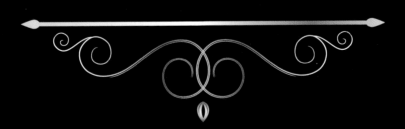

You guessed it. I don't believe there are any hard and fast rules when it comes to sex, any more than there are for any other area of life. A bad bitch should feel free to enjoy her body any way she wants to. That said, if you master a few tips for getting your guy into the bedroom and pleasing him once you're there, you're bound to have fun and feel empowered, and who doesn't want that? That's why I'm planning to devote plenty of time and energy to helping you all to be bad bitches in the bedroom.

THE ART OF SEDUCTION

People always ask me how I get men to do what I want. My answer is one simple word: *seduction.* Master it, and you'll have them eating out of the palm of your hand. This is actually quite a challenge, because it requires tremendous confidence and steady poise, but we've been working up to the big reveal, and I know you're ready, ladies.

In a world where we dress sexy, talk sexy, and text sexy, one of the most seductive means of getting a man's attention isn't particularly sexy at all. Gently rubbing someone's arm or leg can be way more enticing than being provocative or actually getting naked. I'm serious. If you sit across from a man and gaze right into his eyes with that certain look—you know the one—and then touch his leg or arm, he'll be completely yours. Honestly, I've found that's the best way to seduce a man. Plus, as much as I'm all for letting men be men and take the lead when it comes to dating and sex, I think most guys like getting that little sign from us that shows we're 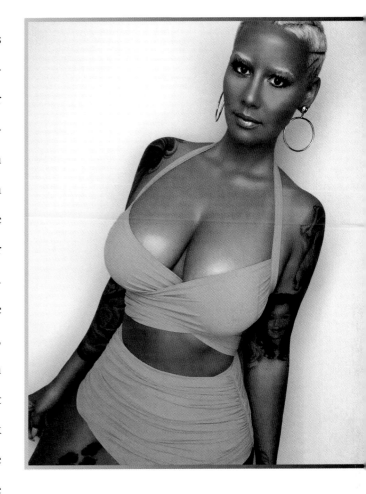 interested, so they can make their move. I think it can even be cute for a girl to be a little bit forward in showing a guy she likes him. As long as you don't go overboard and you maintain that classy bad-bitch attitude we've been practicing all along, a little flirtation—or even making the first move—can really catch a guy's attention.

Don't be afraid to compliment the man you like, either. Think about how good compliments make you feel. Men also love that feeling. Many women don't do this, maybe because they're afraid of being too forward. I say, take the risk. Life's too short not to go for what you want, and being confident is always sexy. Pick out something unexpected. Obviously, if he has gorgeous eyes, don't just go for that. Instead, compliment something most people wouldn't notice.

He'll maybe blush and say, "Shit. Thanks." But I can tell he loves it.

SMIZE

If you've ever watched the TV show *America's Next Top Model,* you've seen Tyra Banks working her magic, teaching her girls how to make an impact with one simple expression: the smize. What she really means is to smile with your eyes. If you want something from someone—whether it's a job or a kiss—make him want to give it to you. To do so, you should create a feeling of connection by drawing him in with a smile that conveys warmth and power. Master that stare, and you can make any man blush, no matter how strong he is, how famous he is, or how much money he has. Once you've got it down, you can literally lock in any man. It's a stare that will give any man a hard-on in a second. It's going to make him think, *Fuck, this girl, there's something about her. There's something I need to know about her. There's something so sexy and seductive about her. I can't quite put my finger on it.*

You're not licking your lips. You're not even being particularly sexual. You're just being subtly provocative and very, very present. Your eyes lock with his, and it's like everything else around you doesn't even matter. You're telling him with your eyes, *That hot guy over there, I know he's there, but I'm not paying him any mind. I'm looking right at you.* Think about how you look at someone you're deeply in love with, as if he's perfect, almost godlike. It's that same type of stare. It's that same type of energy.

Seduction is almost like a dance. You want to get something out of a man—sex or love or money. He wants to get something from you in exchange, so you give him the impression of closeness or attraction or sex or whatever else it is he wants. But of course, now he wants more from you. And so you have to stay one step ahead of him, keeping him interested without giving away more than you're willing to lose. A man always wants a little bit more, and you're always one move ahead, keeping him interested. When it's working, it's the best feeling in the world. But no joke, this is some next-level bad-bitch behavior. Not for beginners or amateurs. You've got to

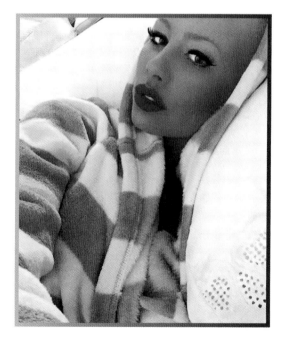

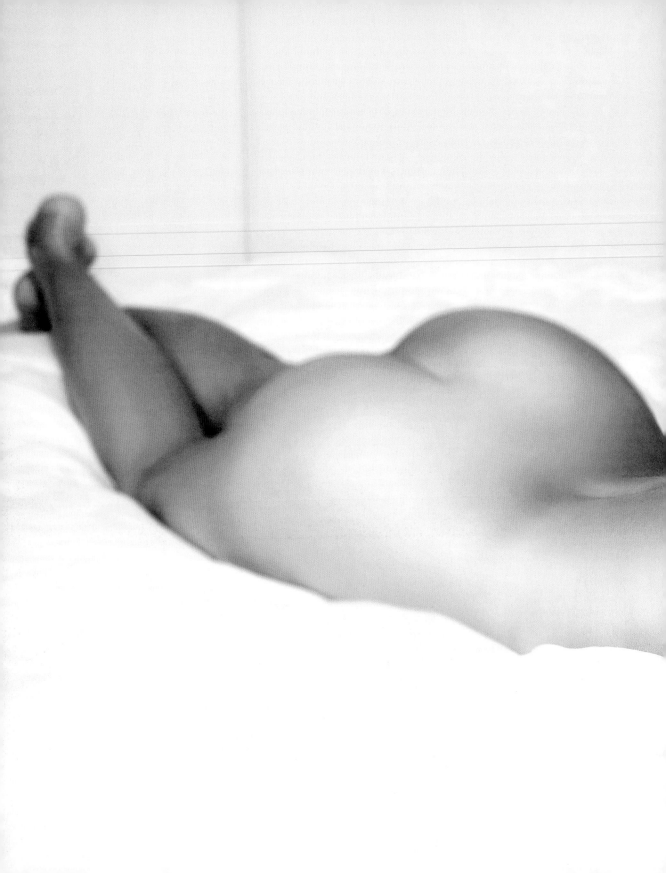

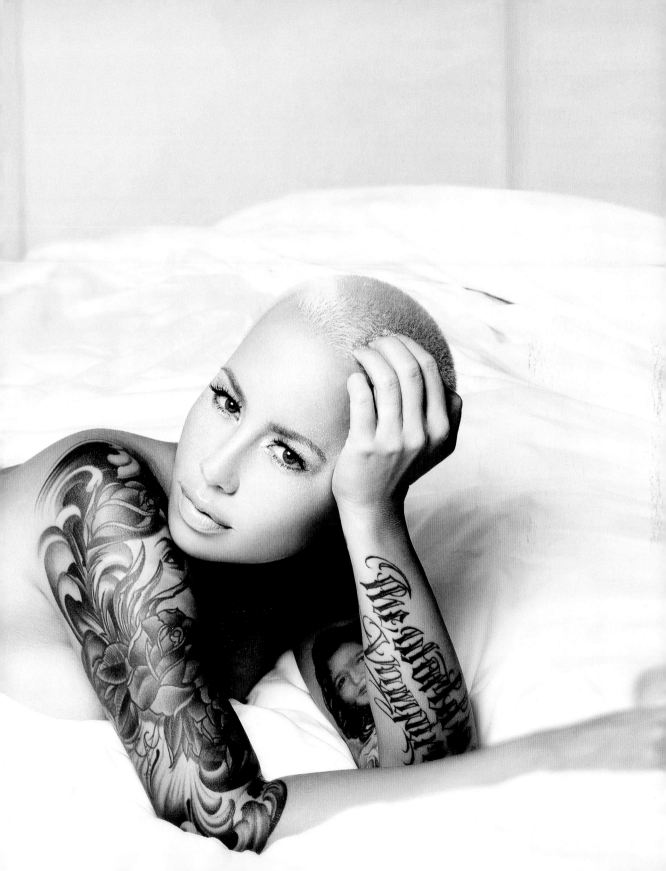

have every other aspect of yourself together before you can attempt to lure someone in.

IN THE MOOD

If the guy you like is coming over, definitely groom yourself. Do whatever it is you do to feel sexy. Put on some nice indoor makeup. You don't need the works—after all, if you're planning on going to bed, you don't want to look crazy afterward. Go with a nice little lash, lip gloss, and blush. That's plenty.

Now, to get him in the mood—and let him know you're in the mood—there are definitely some subtle moves you can make. Just don't go overboard. You don't want to give off the vibe that you're some horny porn star (unless you are, in which case he already knows, and more power to you). If a guy you're just starting to see comes over and you've got sex books and toys everywhere, he might be into it, but he might be totally weirded out.

I don't think there's anything wrong with having some drinks available. You don't want to get wasted and potentially do something you'll regret, but sharing a nice bottle of wine is sweet and seductive. Candlelight is always romantic, as are dimmed lights. You want to set the mood with finesse and grace—it shouldn't look like he's coming over just to have sex with you. (Unless it really is a booty call. And you know what I'll say to that: You go, girl.)

All About Oral

I think sometimes girls get intimidated by blow jobs because they don't really know what to do, or they haven't figured out how to enjoy it, and so it becomes a chore. That's not fun for anyone. It's not fun for the girls, and it's not fun for the guys, either. My best advice is just to relax and stop overthinking it. The biggest hurdle I've heard for most girls is worrying about looking ugly while doing something that, honestly, can be kind of unattractive. A girl spends her whole life trying to be pretty, and then she finally gets a guy's interest, and he wants her to do something that's going to make her gag and drool and make her eyes pop out of her head. The thing is, that's not what the guy is thinking about right then. At all. Put yourself in his shoes: You're hooking up with a *hot* girl. Would *you* really be thinking about that?

Sometimes guys will make it clear they want oral sex. But when they don't, and if it's something you're angling to do, then I say go ahead and make it happen—without being totally inappropriate, of course. In my experience, most guys will find your willingness super-sexy. If you're enjoying yourself, it will always be better for the guy. And so I think it's OK to be sexually proactive—within reason—and to be the one who makes it happen.

It's not all about him, though. Oral sex should be good for you, too. If you're on the receiving end, and the guy doesn't know what he's doing, here's a sweet, sexy way to teach him what's up. Grab his hand, and lick the soft pocket of skin between his thumb and pointer finger in order to show him exactly how you want it. Not only is that a turn-on for him, but you'll be more likely to get exactly what you want. You shouldn't be afraid to tell him what to lick or not to lick and what to touch or not to touch.

I think it's OK to be sexually proactive—within reason—and to be the one who makes it happen.

Don't be afraid to speak up about your likes and dislikes. You know what I hate? When a guy grabs your head and pushes it down onto his crotch. It's annoying, and it's disrespectful. When you're already there, it can be sexy, but if you're in the middle of a pre-hookup conversation, that's wack. Let me want to do it, dude. Don't make me feel obligated or pressured, especially if I'm not into it.

At first, you want to keep it light and sexy, even if you don't like what he's doing. Turn your annoyances into jokes, and he should get the hint. "Don't grab my head like that, because then I'll grab your head and make you do what I want *you* to do." If he still isn't getting the picture or honoring your comfort zones, you've got to cut him loose. I mean, do you really want to be doing something you hate with someone who's clueless for the rest of your life?

DIFFERENT STROKES FOR DIFFERENT FOLKS

Beyond a few tips, it's hard to compile a list of do's and don'ts, because people are into so many different things. There's stuff one woman will do and enjoy, while another woman is like "absolutely not." Find out what your man likes in bed and make sure he gets it, without doing anything that makes you uncomfortable. You don't need to play around. Just ask him what he likes, straight up.

Here's the thing. Most guys like it dirty. Honestly, so many guys love a classy lady who can be a nasty freak in the bedroom, rather than yet another girl who's just lying on her back. I think guys do get nervous, even if they act like they don't. They want to know you're into it and that it's fun for you. Sex is a big part of a relationship, for sure. And there's nothing to be embarrassed about if you think a particular activity is sexy, too. I've heard guys talking about being into all different kinds of stuff, from spitting into a girl's mouth to shooting cum onto her face. If you're into it, go for it. If you're giving a blow job and you don't want to swallow, get him to give you a facial instead. Guys love the money shot.

I personally prefer a man who makes a lot of noise in the bedroom.

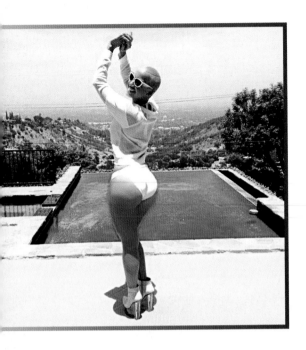

That way, I know exactly what feels good for him. That's very important to me, and it turns me on. But if a guy's quiet, I don't automatically kick him to the curb. I think there are ways to talk about everything, really. Do your best to keep it light and make it sexy. Say something like "I want to hear you. Talk to me." I think most guys are also into a girl who's vocal. If you feel shy or you're not comfortable talking dirty, you can definitely respond with facial expressions and moaning or breathing heavy. That'll turn a guy on quickly. You're there having sex with them, so he knows you want to have sex. Now he just wants to know you're enjoying it.

The best way to make sure you're turned on while turning him on is to be sure you don't go to bed with anyone you're not really into. Then, while it's happening, let it flow. Don't be so worried about what comes next or whether he wants to take your relationship to the next level. Just have fun.

If there's something you're genuinely not into, don't lie and pretend you are. It's just like how at the beginning of a relationship, you're not going to say you like to cook if you don't. When you're first sleeping with someone new, if you pretend to like something you don't, it's going to be harder to voice that dislike later.

Life Happens

Sex is full of potentially mortifying moments, especially when you're first sleeping with a new guy and you're still getting comfortable with each other. But, really and truly, try not to worry about it too much. I know some girls get embarrassed when they queef, but you just can't sweat it. Any mature man can handle it. Guys are way less uptight about, well, pretty much everything than girls are, and they don't give a fuck about that kind of nonsense. I'd say just ignore the fact that it happened, because it'll probably happen again, and keep on doing what you're doing. If stuff like that isn't happening, then you probably aren't having really good, raunchy sex anyhow.

Oh, while we're on the topic of how girls see the world versus how guys do, girls worry about cellulite way more than guys do. Guys don't care. All girls, even skinny minnies, have cellulite. If guys minded, they wouldn't be with women at all. If a guy doesn't like it, fuck him. That's just how God made us.

There's only so much you can plan in advance when you're getting ready to go to bed with a new guy. In the end, it all comes down to chemistry. And if you thought you liked a guy only to find out you have bad chemistry, make up an excuse and get out. Seriously, life's too short. Say you have a dentist appointment or a family engagement in the morning. Of course, if he just does one thing you don't like, try talking to him or showing him another way. But if it's all bad from the beginning, that's no good.

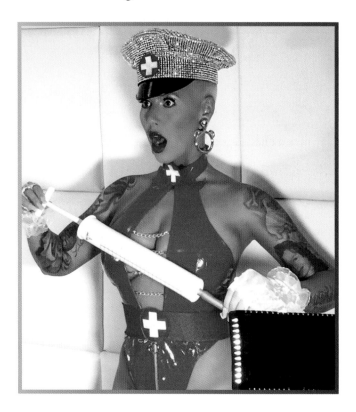

Years ago, I went on a date with a guy, and it was really cool. He was good-looking, and we were having a good time. Then, at the end of our date, I found out we had totally awful sexual chemistry, right from the get-go. We kissed, and he started biting at my mouth. Seriously, his teeth were all over me. And the next day, my mouth was all cut up. It totally canceled out our great date. I never spoke to him again. There's nothing worse than a bad kisser. Well, actually there is: biting me up. It was fucking weird.

To Fuck or Not to Fuck

Yes, you should be free to have sex with anyone you want, as long as he's not in another relationship and neither are you. But there are ways to be smart about it that can save you a lot of grief down the road. If you know a group of guys who are all friends, or even just run in the same circles, don't sleep with more than one of them. You want to maintain your reputation, and there are plenty of men out there.

Also, don't ever sleep with a guy because you feel you should or you feel you have to in order to make him like you. The thing with guys—and it's the same with girls, really—is that they love a challenge. In general, I think girls worry way too much about making people—especially guys—like them. Of course, be feminine and flirty and fun. But don't be afraid to be a real person, which means you're allowed to have opinions or want something different from what he wants. If you're sweet all the way around, he's likely to take advantage of you. It's good to have a tough side, too. That's why my motto is "MILF, sweetheart, badass." I'm a little bit of everything, and it's a good balance. Find your own particular balance, and you'll find a guy who's just right for you.

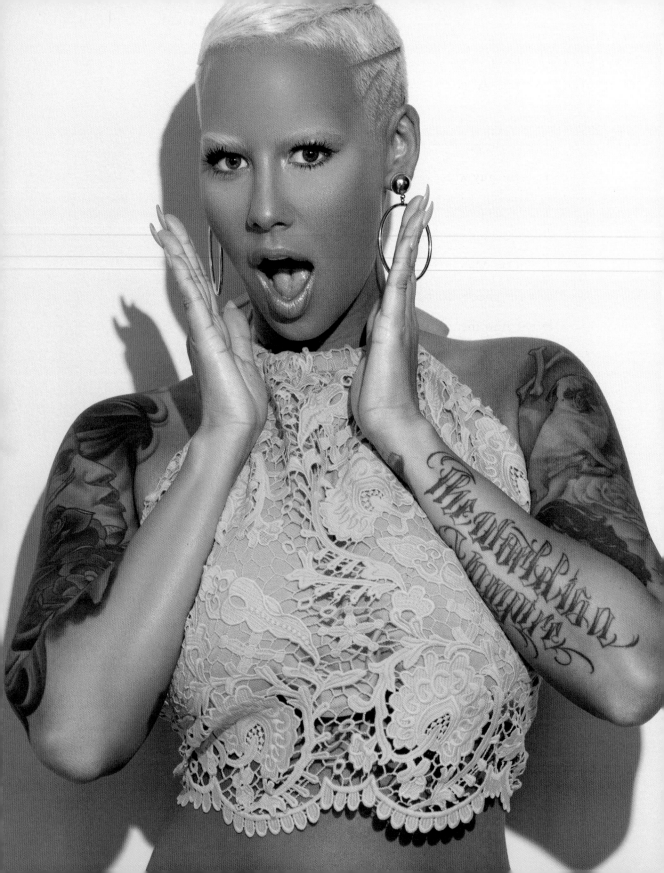

When a bad bitch gets busy in the bedroom, she always uses condoms. And if the guy won't agree? Then tell him to go fuck himself. Especially nowadays, there's just too much out there not to be safe. You don't want to have raw sex with someone who's not committed to you. I know condoms suck. Many girls are sensitive to latex. Listen, I am, too. But condoms are a necessary precaution, and you have to use them. I always do. Always. And there are alternatives to latex. Polyurethane is just as effective for protecting against pregnancy, and it is more pleasurable for some people. But they do break more easily, so always be on point. Lambskin condoms are also available, but they don't protect against STDs, so don't even go there.

Once you're in a relationship, you can take it to the next level by saying something like "Let's go get tested together." But that's only if you both make a commitment to each other and you both want to be in a monogamous relationship. Even then, you should still always use a condom. But then, one night, if you get caught up in the passion and love you feel for each other, you'll know you're most likely safe.

At the end of the day, if you want to fuck a guy, do it. Don't expect him to marry you, although he could. I'm just saying, don't feel bad if he doesn't. Don't feel ashamed of your desire, either, because guess what? Men go out and get some all the time, without anyone making a fuss about it. It's not our problem that there's a double standard in our culture. We should be free to do what we want, just like men are. That's why the character of Samantha from *Sex and the City* is so empowering. She wasn't some dirty whore; she was a bad bitch who loved sex, and she wasn't ashamed of it. The easiest thing in the world is to get a guy to sleep with you, because a guy will stick his dick in a block of Swiss cheese.

So if it's a mutual attraction and you want an easy lay, that's OK. Just don't expect too much. And, just because you had sex with a guy, that doesn't mean he fully conquered you. As long as you take care of yourself—don't make it weird, become clingy, call him every five minutes, or try to make him your boyfriend all of a sudden—it could simply be a fun fling. It's up to you to remember that casual sex is exactly that. If you're clear on that going into it, you shouldn't feel bad about anything you choose to do or get your heart broken. In fact, ladies, think about it

We should be free to do what we want, just like men are.

this way: not every guy you sleep with is actually worthy of being your boyfriend (if that's your thing). It's one thing to have a one-night stand, but don't be ready and willing to rush out and give away your heart so easily.

Have a little self-respect. If you show him that you do, he's definitely more likely to respect you, too. Many times, when a guy sleeps with a girl, he might like her because she's cute and it was fun. But if he's going to be her boyfriend, he'll have to know her better. What's she like? Is she going to be cool with his friends? Is she going to want the same things out of life that he does? Sometimes a woman gets her feelings hurt if a guy she had a one-night stand with never calls her again. When, really, we ladies should be applying the same logic to our sex life. A guy shouldn't expect a rela-

tionship from you if you've casually slept with him. And if you're not into that idea, don't sleep around. Remember, you've always got to think of yourself first.

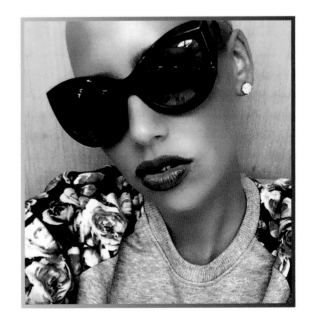

The day after you hook up with someone, of course, you want him to text you. That's totally natural. We all feel that way (unless it was really awful or he turned out to be a creep). But picking up your phone every five seconds to see if he did isn't going to make it any more likely to happen. This is when all of your bad-bitch training really comes into play. You're too busy and fabulous to let your life get derailed by a man. Instead, you ought to take care of what you've got to do that day.

I know this can be so hard to do. It's human nature to get worked up about this kind of stuff. And many women are emotional creatures who find it very difficult to be logical about it. If you start feeling insecure, that's when your girlfriends can be lifesavers. Complain as much as you want, but no matter what advice they give you, don't cave. Don't text him. Know your worth. If a guy does care, he's going to reach out to you, for sure. If he doesn't, then it's better to know now, before you really start to fall for him. And life's too short to get hung up on one night with one guy you didn't even really know all that well yet.

BE COOL

If you have sex with a guy and he wants to leave right away or gets up at the crack of dawn to sneak out, don't stress about it. Whatever he wants to do, let him do it. You definitely don't want to say, "Stay." And then have him say, "Nah." That's not good. And whatever you do, don't beg. Have some pride, girl. Some guys leave before breakfast. Some guys stay for the entire next day. It doesn't necessarily mean anything either way.

If you go out again, you can tell him later that you would have liked it if he'd stayed. And if you don't, then maybe it's better that you didn't spend more time with him and get attached. If someone's going to like you or you're going to like him, it will happen, no matter what. And you never know why he left. He might be giving you your space. He might have had to work. He might literally have had a dentist appointment. Don't feel bad about it.

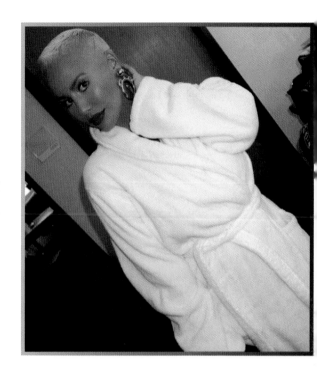

A Bad Bitch Finds Her Own Man

A bad bitch *never* messes with another woman's man. Never. Hell, no. A bad bitch always has her own man. She's never a home wrecker. She doesn't ever knowingly have sex or get into a relationship with a man who's already in a relationship. If you find out after you've already slept with a man that he's in a relationship, you now have the opportunity to end it with him right away. And then move on. It's not your responsibility to tell the other woman. You don't know what's going on in their relationship.

It could be that he just made a mistake and they'll actually get through this, and if there's a chance of that, you don't want to be the one to make it impossible. And if he is a dog, she'll find out eventually. If she does find out somehow and you end up in the middle of their nightmare, apologize to the other woman. Let her know that you had no idea they were together. Be the bigger person, and be super-apologetic. She will obviously be very emotional in that moment, and you'll want to treat her with as much kindness as you'd want to receive in the same situation. Whether she finds out or not, you absolutely should not see him anymore. You're better than that.

TURNING IT AROUND

Maybe you realize after you had sex with a guy that it was a mistake. You had a little too much to drink or you got carried away, and you went farther than you'd intended to at the start of the night. Fear not. There are definitely ways to turn it around.

If you actually like the guy, it's still possible that you might be able to pursue a relationship. First of all, he has to reach out to you. If he doesn't, it's over before it started. If he does, let him know it was spur-of-the-moment with him because it just felt right. Don't make too big a deal of it. Depending on his response, you'll know at that point if he just wants you as a fuck buddy or if he wants to pursue something real with you.

If he did call you back and he's into the idea of going out with you on another date, this is basically your one and only chance at a clean slate. Whatever you do, don't sleep with him again (no matter how good the sex was—if you play it right, there's much more where that came from).

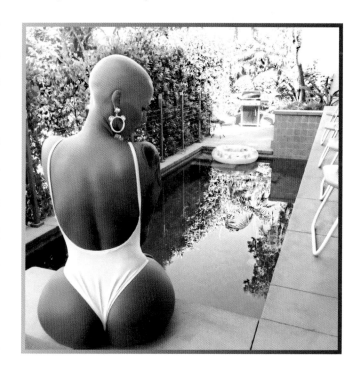

If you realize after the fact that you're actually not interested in him, it's important to be strong and not sleep with him again. Don't be drunk-dialing him or whatever. Or if you do, just know that he's probably going to start thinking you really do like him, and it's going to get complicated. If you booty-call someone, make sure he knows it's a booty call. And never booty-call someone who likes you. That's a recipe for disaster—for him and for you.

Never, ever send nude photos to a guy. When I say never, I mean fucking *never*. If you do and then you break up, you'll have anxiety for the rest of your life about whether he's going to put that shit out in social media. It's one thing to post seductive, partially naked photos online, with full consciousness of what you're doing and an awareness that the whole world is potentially going to see them. But when a guy texts you and asks you for a naked picture, just think of your kids, your parents, your family, everyone who could possibly see it on the Internet if he decides to leak it. It's not

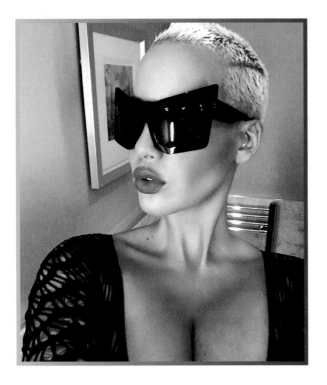

worth it. You might think it's OK to send a shot that doesn't include your face, but you could still be identified by your tattoos or other unique characteristics. If you absolutely have to send something, then do a sexy shot of your face and cleavage. That's plenty. No nudes. No body shots. Trust me, I learned the hard way. If he wants to see you naked that badly, he can make the effort to come see you in the flesh.

On the other hand, I don't think there's anything wrong with sexting. You just have to know when the time is right and how far to go. I'd advise letting him take the lead, as long as you stop when you're about to jump out of your comfort zone. But if the guy's clearly into it and you're into it, then it can be really fun. And it can give you an opportunity to tell him what you're into. You can also ask him what he likes. That way, when it comes time to have sex, you'll know how to please him.

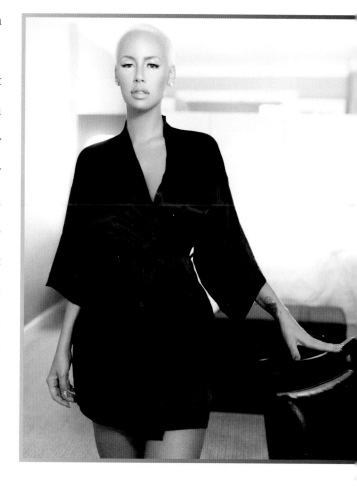

The only hard and fast rule is to always be yourself and only do what you feel comfortable with. If you have to do anything other than that to keep him interested, he's not worth it. Sex is supposed to be fun and make you feel good. You're a bad bitch, remember? You don't settle for anything that's not making you happy in any area of your life and certainly not in the bedroom.

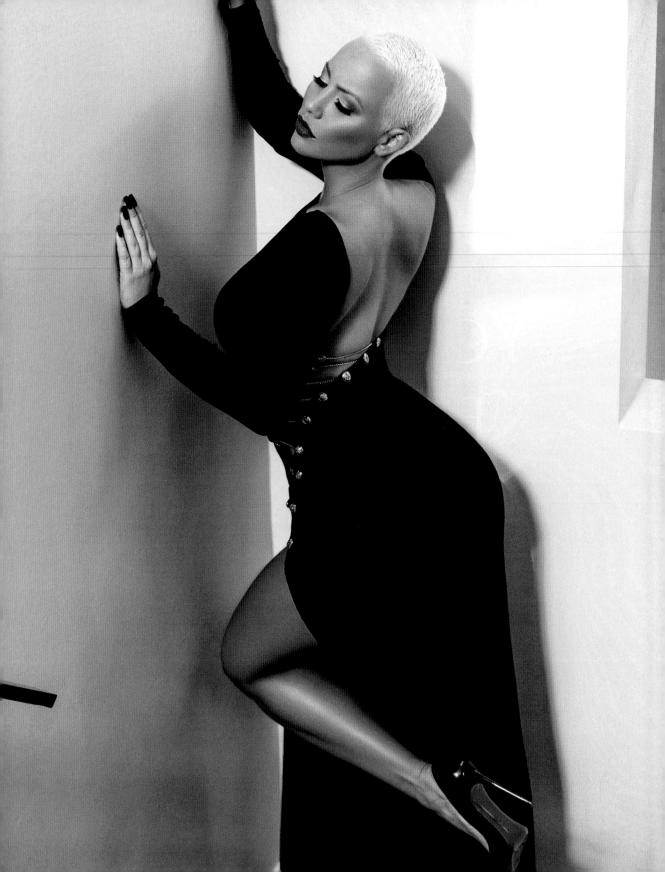

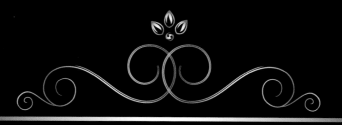

12

You Can't Keep a Bad Bitch Down:
Evolve or Die

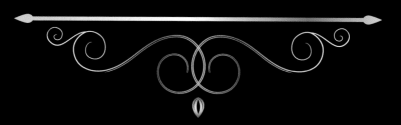

No matter how strong you are and how hard you work it, life isn't always going to go your way. Friends flake. Breakups happen. Businesses fall apart. Marriages end. Sometimes you're even the one who had to weigh the pros and cons and make the break. How a bad bitch deals with the dark days is just as important as how she deals with the good ones. Not only does hardship make us stronger, but it also helps us grow. Something that feels shitty at the time may actually end up being a blessing because it takes us to where we're really meant to be in our lives. Setbacks and learning how to deal with them reveal meaningful sides of ourselves along the way.

Make Yourself an Even Badder Bitch

Not only should you not wallow and let yourself go, but you should also make yourself better. Don't sit in your house, eating and gaining weight. Instead, this is your time to hit the gym, get your hair done, maybe do a little shopping for yourself. Invest in making yourself an even badder bitch than you ever were before. Use all of your anger and passion to fuel your makeover. This is also a great time to reevaluate your original vision and ask yourself if it's still working for you. Maybe you're moving on to a new stage of your life, and that means reinventing your look, your career, or the way you spend your time. Whatever you envision you can create. You've already proven this to yourself during all the steps you took to become a bad bitch. I know it may be frustrating to feel like you're starting back at square one. But you're really not doing that. No matter what's going on in your life right now, no one and nothing can take away all that you've accomplished to get here. Now you just have to redouble your efforts, and you'll achieve even more. You'll see! Before you know it, you'll meet another guy, get another job, or get back on top. Then you'll have the power to decide what you want and when. You'll be able to choose how to live your life and with whom.

It's Our World, and We Rule It

We've spent a lot of time talking about how to be the baddest bitches we can be in the world we live in now, but I want to leave you with an even more powerful thought. Not only do we have the opportunity to respond to our current place in society with grace and strength and to achieve as much abundance and love and pleasure as we want, but we can also take it one step further. We can actually make a stand for what we believe in and

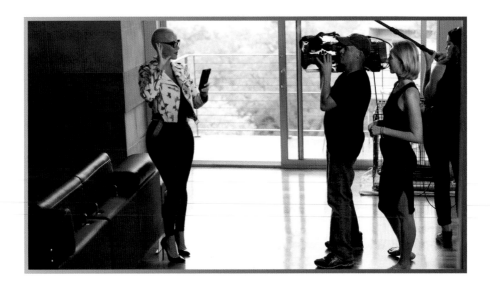

start reinventing the space around us. The world we live in is typically represented as a woman, Mother Earth, so why not make her a bad bitch, too?

It's time for us to come into our full power, ladies. I just led a seminar for a bunch of female college students in Detroit, and they asked me some questions that made me realize how passionate I am about my bad-bitch mission, just how crucial it is, and just how far I intend to go with it. After I was done telling my whole story and talking about why slut-shaming is bad and we shouldn't do it, and how we can all be powerful women, I opened up the floor to questions.

One young woman raised her hand to speak. "Because it's a man's world, as women, even if we want to be powerful, we have to look and act a certain way to get men to hire us."

I understood what she saw around her to make her think like this, but I was about to set the record straight for her. "One, it is not a man's world,"

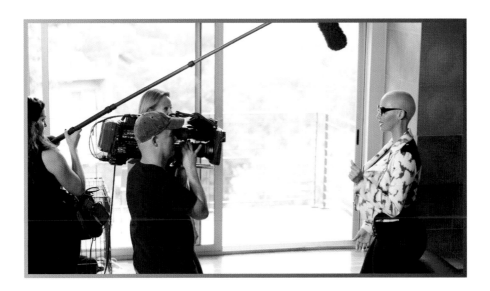

I said. "Two, the reason I'm here talking to you girls is so you can be the CEO of your own company and not need to ask any man for a job. And three, you don't have to conform to society's standards of what you should wear. You can wear whatever the fuck you want. If you're trying to get a job at an office, maybe you shouldn't wear a tiny skirt and midriff top, but that has nothing to do with living in a man's world. You dress for what you want in life."

I shared my message with this group of young women at this college, and I'll say it to all of you. We have the power. We do. But we have to own it. We have to be on point with our behavior in all aspects of our life, so no one can say no to us for any reason. And when they do try to hold us back or make us doubt ourselves, we have to support one another to come back stronger than ever, again and again, until there's no way we can be denied by the doubters or haters or anyone who thought they could disrespect us.

A Bad Bitch Always Ends Up on Top

No matter what your difficulty may be, you'll end up on top eventually. In fact, you'll be better off than you ever were before. Don't doubt it for a second, no matter how low you may feel sometimes. Anything that forces you to be stronger, no matter how painful it is, only makes you better. And that can only help you be a badder bitch. Even when it takes awhile, a bad bitch always gets her way, by any means necessary.

So no matter what happens in your life, remember this: A bad bitch is strong. She is powerful. She is fierce. She is intelligent. She is honest. She is loving. She lives with integrity, and she shares her beauty and light while changing the world. **She is you.**

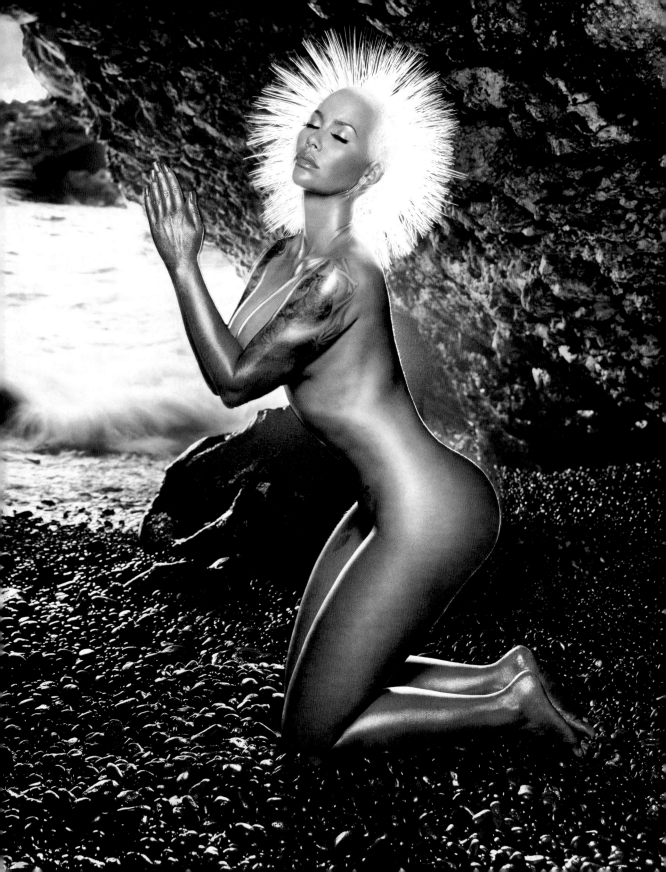

ACKNOWLEDGMENTS

Sebastian, you are my light. You have brought so much joy into my life. You're mommy's little pumpkin.

To *my dad*, thank you for being stern with me growing up. A young girl always needs that.

My little brothers, *Mikey and Brian*, I love you.

Donna Norris, you've always been like the sister I never had. Thank you for always keeping my swag up when I couldn't afford to on my own.

Priscilla Ono, you're my best friend. Thank you for always being there for me and making me look beautiful.

Thank you, *Walter Mosley*, for being one of my best friends, and for being like my big brother and handling my business like I really am your sister. You're one of the smartest guys I know.

A big thank-you to *Nick Cannon* for giving me the opportunity to meet with Simon & Schuster and make this book happen.

A special thanks to *Jen Bergstrom* and everyone at Simon & Schuster for letting me fully express myself and be creative while writing this book.

Thank you to *Nina Cordes* and *Jeremie Ruby-Strauss* at Gallery for all their hard work to make this book possible.

David LaChapelle, you are truly a creative genius. You brought my book to life with your photography.

Special thanks to my team, *Benji, Joseph, Tia, Cordell, Will, Brendan Forbes,* and *Sarah Tomlinson*. You guys help me, every day, to become a better person.

PHOTO CREDITS

Page 113: Courtesy of the author

Pages 114–15: Photo by Brendan Forbes

Pages 116 and 118: Courtesy of the author

Page 120: Photo by David LaChapelle

Pages 123, 124, 126, 129, 130, 132, 136, 139, 141, 142: Courtesy of the author

Page 143: Courtesy of Dottie Rose

Page 145: Courtesy of the author

Page 146: Photo by Brendan Forbes

Pages 151, 152, 156, 158, 159: Courtesy of the author

Page 161: Courtesy of Dottie Rose

Page 162: Photo by Brendan Forbes

Page 166: Courtesy of the author

Pages 168, 170–171: Photos by Brendan Forbes

Page 173 and 174: Courtesy of the author

Page 177: Courtesy of the author

Page 178: Photo by Brendan Forbes

Page 184: Courtesy of the author

Page 188–189: Photo by Brendan Forbes

Pages 193 and 194: Courtesy of the author

Page 196: Courtesy of Dottie Rose

Pages 198–199: Photo by Brendan Forbes

Pages 200, 202, 203: Courtesy of the author

Page 204: Photo by David LaChapelle

Page 207: Photo by Brendan Forbes

Page 209: Courtesy of the author

Pages 210–211: Photo by Brendan Forbes

Pages 216 and 218: Courtesy of the author

Page 220: Photo by Brendan Forbes

Pages 223, 225, 227, 228: Courtesy of the author

Pages 229 and 230: Photos by Brendan Forbes

Pages 234 and 235: Courtesy of the author

Page 237: Photo by David LaChapelle